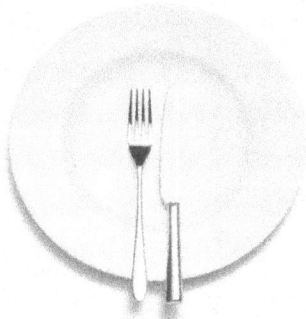

FOOD

SENSE AND REASON

DISCLAMER
This book provides general information only. It is based on information gathered from a large number of different sources. It does not provide any form of medical advice and it is not a substitute for the advice of your own doctor, medical practitioner or health care professional. Readers are specifically advised to consult their doctor regarding the treatment of any medical condition that they have. The author of this book shall not be held liable or responsible for any misuse or misunderstanding of the information contained in this book or for any loss, damage or injury caused or alleged to be caused either directly or indirectly by any action that is consequential to reading the contents of this book.
No part of this book has been evaluated or approved by any medical, scientific, professional or Food or Drug Administration Authority.

Contents

Introduction

It is an undisputed fact that over the last sixty years the health of people living in the western world has deteriorated and it is continuing to do so at an alarming rate. Millions die each year from health problems that are totally preventable. As our wealth and affluence increased our health declined and we are now facing an epidemic of chronic diseases that are close to overwhelming our health care systems.

It is also an undisputed fact that around the world levels of obesity are rising and today more people are overweight than under nourished. Just about everyone working in the field of health and nutrition agree that our weight, and in particular obesity, is the common link in the decline in our health. The heavier and fatter we become the more our health deteriorates. Whether we like it or not, the bottom line is that we are eating more than our bodies need, the old *"calories in and calories consumed"* conundrum, something that we have been told for years. But are we actually eating more calories than we need? Is the real truth that we are eating too much of the wrong things and not enough of the right things? What ever the truth of the matter, the tragedy is that most of us are unaware of what is happening to us. Worse still, some of the food that many of us eat every day of our lives is not just making us put on weight, it is also damaging our health and leaving us with a legacy of illness and disease in our old age.

"You are what you eat" is an old adage. If we look back into only recent history it is clear that both our lifestyle and our eating habits have changed dramatically. Lack of exercise, snacking between meals, 'TV dinners', fast food and 'super sized' portions are all taking their toll on our health. But are these the only reasons? Are diet and lack of exercise alone causing the problem? Fifty years ago in the United States one in nine adults would have been considered as being obese. Today the worst estimates are that one in four adults are not just overweight, they are actually obese. In developed countries like the UK, America and Australia you often see claims that around two thirds of the adult population is now overweight, and being overweight can quickly lead to obesity. If these figures are correct our waist lines have grown enormously in a very short space of time.

In the developed countries of the western world weight and health problems affect old and young alike. Children are becoming increasingly at risk simply because they inherit the poor diets and eating habits of their parents. It is a well recognised fact that overweight mothers have larger babies that become overweight children and then overweight adults.

The association between our diet, our weight and our health attracts a tremendous amount of media coverage with newspapers, TV programmes and online web sites quick to latch on to the latest fad and celebrity diets. Eat a plant based diet, stop eating meat, go sugar free, eat like a caveman, give up grains and cereals. The list is endless. All of these diets come with a promise of health benefits or weight loss. Hardly a week goes by without some news about food hitting the headlines. Super foods are one of the most recent crazes but more often than not, rather than the food that we should be eating, this news comes as 'scares' that tell us that something we thought was good for us is now bad. How often do we see the phrase "research suggests that" used to qualify unsubstantiated health benefits or the dangers of eating specific types of food. Being economical with the facts and selling miss information or 'Fake News' is nothing new. We listen to the TV and radio broadcasts, search out the web sites and read the books with great enthusiasm but with so much conflicting information we end up feeling very confused. Often it is years later that the full analysis of the research on which the reports are based becomes available, by which time we have changed our eating habits and stopped eating something that is actually quite good for us. The triumph of vegetable oil and margarine as being a healthier option than saturated fat and butter is a classical example of this.

The diet and health food industry is a multi billion dollar business. Despite some very convincing advertising that makes claims to the contrary, meal replacements, supplements and low fat 'skinny' options are not the solution when it comes to eating a healthy diet or losing weight. In fact the vast majority of diet products go against the basic principles of good nutrition and are not only bad for our health, they also make us feel hungry so we end up eating more. Does 'dieting' work? Received wisdom tells us that if you eat less and get more exercise you will lose weight. Well there are very few of us who can honestly say that at some time in their life they have not 'been on a diet' but how many of us have lost weight and then managed to keep that weight off? Very few. Most of us put it back on and end up in a vicious circle of yo-yo dieting that usually involves counting calories and the consumption of diet products. It is hardly surprising that the word 'diet' conjures up images of deprivation, feeling hungry and being miserable. So if a 'diet' is going to work it needs to be doable, sustainable and enjoyable, something that you can do for the rest of your life.

No matter what your age or state of health it is never too late to start eating a healthy diet and a healthy diet should not take the fun out of eating. But what is a healthy diet? In a world where healthy eating has become shrouded in myths and misinformation most of us struggle to find the answer. With so much confusion around do we simply no longer know how to eat what is good for us?

Strange as it may seem, when it comes to a healthy diet there is no one size fits all. We have been programmed by nature to be different and one of the amazing facts about human beings is that we are able to adapt to our environment and find a meal almost anywhere. We have evolved to survive. There is no doubt that some food is good to eat, some food is not quite so good and some food is actually quite bad, so understanding the 'what' and the 'why' of healthy eating is key to being able to make informed decisions about the food you eat and finding the diet that is right for you.

So why did we change our eating habits and why is some of the food we are eating close to being a ticking bomb when it comes to our health?

Well in the early 1970's snack foods first appeared and we were seduced by major advertising campaigns into snacking between meals. In the mid 1980's super sized portions came on the scene and as food generally became cheaper we could afford to buy more and eat more. But while all this was going on we were being told some serious fibs about food. How and why this happened is anyone's guess. You could be cynical and say it was the food industry feeding us false information. It could have been confused science or scientists getting it wrong because they had a theory to prove, or it could have been journalists only interested in sensational media coverage. Who knows. But the end result is that we believed what we were told and the fibs about food ended up changing eating habits around the world.

Chapter One

You Are What You Eat

You Are What You Eat

"You are what you eat" is an interesting adage but have you ever wondered where it came from? The origin of the phrase is attributed to an early 19th Century French epicure and gastronome named Anthelme Brillat-Savarin who used it in his book *"Physiologie du Gout"*. A book by the way that had nothing to do with the disease gout, translated it means *'The physiology of Taste'*.

In the 1920's and early 1930's an American nutritionist called Victor Lindlahr, who was a strong believer in the idea that the food we eat controls our health, developed the Catabolic Diet. At the time this diet and his views gained some adherents and this led to the earliest known printed example of the saying in an advertisement in the Bridgeport Telegraph in 1923:

"Ninety per cent of the diseases known to man are caused by cheap food stuffs. You are what you eat"

Ironically this advertisement was for beef, a food that with modern factory farming methods is no where near the 'healthy' meat it was then. In 1942 Lindlahr published a book with the title

"You are what you eat; How to win and keep health with diet"

This book appears to be what brought the saying into public awareness. In the 1960's it had a new lease of life when the Hippy culture used it as their slogan for healthy eating.

So are we really what we eat? The interaction between the food we eat and our health is extremely complex. As well as determining what we look like and how susceptible we are to disease, scientists now know that genetics can have a major impact on how our bodies digest and use the food we eat. Much of what we do know about the relationship between diet and health is either the result of population studies undertaken over large numbers of people over periods of several years or laboratory experiments that try hard to mimic the human body. In reality, despite an astoundingly rapid increase in our understanding we still have an lot to learn about the complex inter relationships between our health and the food we eat.

When it comes to understanding and writing about diet, health and nutrition many of us have an unintentional 'hidden agenda' and as a consequence all too often we succumb to a sort of 'tunnel vision' and only see what we want to see. The analysis and use of data can at the end of the day be both selective and subjective.

For centuries some diseases have been closely linked to diet. Gout is one of them and it is also one of the chronic diseases that is now afflicting more and more people. But is it possible that diet alone can cause gout? In horrendous pain my husband was told by an orthopaedic surgeon,

" You're eating too many purines and not drinking enough water. You're 'crispy' "

What's a purine? ·····... Something you eat, it's in your food"

Having been 'children of the swinging sixties' we had always believed that you are what you eat. In fact we thought our diet was quite healthy, so the challenge was to find out whether something we were eating was causing so much pain and distress. Little did I know then that the end result of this seemingly simple question would be a lifelong change in our diet and the shocked realisation that the food that was causing my husband's gout is slowly and insidiously making us all ill. Sadly few of us realise that this is happening, especially as some of the food that is making us ill is actually promoted as the 'healthy option'. Horrendously painful it may be, but for the gout sufferer gout is in reality a wake up call because it is giving you a clear message that your body is not working properly. Did the gout go away? Yes, and contrary to received wisdom that says once you have gout you will have it for life, it has stayed away.

So what has our modern diet got to do with gout and the other chronic diseases that are increasing at such an alarming rate? Well in order to understand this we first need some science. If you are up to speed on your human biology skip to Chapter Two, if not read on.

The Building Blocks

The human body is a highly complex organism that contains around 10 trillion cells. It is a massive biological engine that is fuelled by the food we eat, the water we drink and the air we breathe. In the cells that make up our bodies thousands of different biochemical reactions are taking place each second, breaking down and converting food, water and oxygen into the energy we need and the compounds that make up our bodies.

For all living things food is essential. Without it they ultimately die. But what is it in food that our bodies need? What happens to food when we eat and digest it? Why is eating different types of food important? And how does the food we eat provide the fuel our bodies need? Why can't we live on leaves and fruit like our close relatives the chimpanzees? If you have ever asked yourself any of these questions then read on. You will begin to understand how amazing our bodies are and why 'You really are what you eat'.

The three key elements of our diet are proteins, carbohydrates and fats, but we also need vitamins, minerals, micro nutrients, trace elements, fibre and water. Together these provide us not only with the energy we need to 'keep us alive' they also provide the enormous number of different materials that our body needs to keep our immune system in good order and repair or replace damaged or dead cells. Just about all of the chemical reactions that take place in our body are helped along and regulated by enzymes and hormones. Our body contains thousands of different ones and each of them is finely tuned to undertake a specific task. Our body switches them on and off as and when it needs them. Without enzymes and hormones it simply will not work. If they become imbalanced things can begin to go wrong. Because just about everything that takes place in our body takes place at the cell level, the first thing to have a basic understanding of are cells.

Cells

Cells are the building blocks of all life on earth. They come in many different shapes and sizes. The 10 trillion cells in the human body are divided into around two hundred different types, each of which perform specific tasks; nerve cells enable us to think and communicate messages to our brains, muscle cells enable us to move and walk about.

They make up our skin, hair, teeth and the haemoglobin in our blood that transports the oxygen we breath around our bodies. All of these cells need energy in order to perform these tasks.

In comparison to other organisms human cells are relatively large and highly complex, but their basic structure and the way in which they work is the same as simple single cell life forms like bacteria. The cell of a bacterium has an outer layer, a cell membrane, that holds the cell together. Inside this membrane is some gel like fluid called cytoplasm. This fluid makes up about 70% of the cell, the rest is protein in the form of enzymes that the cell has made, amino acids, molecules of glucose and something called ATP, Adenosine Triphosphate, a molecule that provides the energy the cell needs to perform its tasks. In the middle of the cell is a single strand of DNA which is coiled into a tight ball, a bit like a ball of string. Molecules of DNA are large and complex and carry the genetic code or blueprint that determines the characteristics of a living thing. It is effectively a sort of 'mission control' of the cell as it holds the pattern that controls just about everything that takes place and in particular the enzymes and hormones that the cell produces.

Human cells have other advanced features and they are far more complex than those of the bacterium but fundamentally they are the same. However, the structure of their DNA is completely different.

DNA, Genes & Chromosomes

The easiest way of understanding DNA, genes and chromosomes is to think of them as being like a strand of glass or plastic beads, with the strand of beads the chromosomes, each of the beads a gene and the DNA the glass or plastic that the beads are made from.

In the centre of each cell in our body there are rod like structures called chromosomes. There are 46 chromosomes in each cell and they are grouped together in 23 pairs. One member of each pair comes from our mother and one member from our father. Twenty two of the pairs are the same for both men and women. The twenty third pair determines our sex and these are called the X and Y chromosomes. Women have two X chromosomes and men have one X and one Y chromosome.

Our genes are made up from DNA and each gene occupies a specific position on a chromosome. With the exception of the X and Y chromosomes there are two copies of each gene. There are approximately 30,000 genes that influence our growth and development.

The DNA is made from four molecules or building blocks called Adenine, Guanine, Cytosine and Thyamine. In the natural living world these four building blocks are found inside the cells of every life form on earth, from simple bacteria to complex multi cell creatures like ourselves. Inside our cells the Adenine, Guanine, Cytosine and Thyamine are combined in different ways and repeated over and over again, in fact three billion times in each set of chromosomes.

As we grow up our bodies duplicate cells by cell division, a process called mitosis. This enables one parent cell to divide into two new daughter cells. However, each day we live some of our cells die, either as a result of damage or as a result of programmed cell death, a process called apoptosis. Interestingly on average between fifty and seventy million cells die each day in a healthy human adult as part of programmed cell death.

Proteins

More or less every function of our body is controlled by proteins. They are the second largest component after water in our body. They form the structural parts of body tissue and our organs and they form part of the DNA that exists in every cell. They also perform a large range of functions in our body, acting as antibodies, enzymes and chemical messengers.

Proteins are made from hundreds and sometimes thousands of smaller units called amino acids. These are held together in long chains to form the protein. Amino acids are classified into twenty different groups. As far as your body is concerned there are two different types of amino acids, some that are essential and some that are non essential. Your body is able to make the non essential amino acids but the essential amino acids, and there are nine in total, cannot be made. The only way we can obtain them is from our food. In order for them to be made 'available' and 'usable' our digestive system breaks proteins down into the amino acids from which they are made. Cells then use the amino acids as building blocks to build enzymes and the structural proteins our body uses. There are between 30,000 and 50,000 different proteins in our body and they are being continuously formed, broken down by enzymes and recycled.

How much protein we need on a daily basis depends on our age and our state of health. On average we need to consume about 0.8 gram of protein for each kilogramme of body weight, so for the 'average' sedentary man this works out at around 56 grams and for a woman 46 grams.

Protein in our diet comes from both animal and vegetable sources. The majority of animal sources, meat, fish, milk and eggs provide us with what is called 'complete protein'. In other words they contain all of the nine essential amino acids. Some vegetable sources like nuts and beans contain complete protein but generally vegetables are low in or missing some of the essential amino acids. However, by combining different vegetables and including nuts and beans in your diet you can obtain all of the essential amino acids you need.

Enzymes

The purpose of an enzyme is to allow a cell to carry out chemical reactions and to carry them out quickly and efficiently. These reactions enable the cell to build things or take things apart as and when needed. As long as a cell's membrane is intact and it is making all of the enzymes it needs to function properly the cell is alive; it is able to create energy from the food we eat, build and maintain its cell wall, reproduce itself and produce new enzymes. At any given time a simple single cell organism contains about a thousand different types of enzymes all working together. The human body contains trillions of cells and each of these cells contain enzymes.

So where do all of these enzymes come from and how does the cell know which enzymes to produce and when to produce them? The answer lies in the cell's DNA. The single strand DNA in a single cell organism like a bacterium is relatively simple but inside human cells we have a much larger and far more sophisticated structure in which short regions of DNA, the genes, define how a specific type of cell works and which enzymes and other compounds it makes.

Enzymes are made from the amino acids that are produced when we digest and breakdown proteins. Because they are made from amino acids the enzymes are themselves also proteins. Each enzyme has a specific size, shape and structure and this defines the specific chemical reaction and, as a consequence, the task that it controls. Without the enzyme the chemical reaction cannot take place. When we digest and breakdown the food we eat our body uses an enormous number of different enzymes;

- carbohydrase and amylase are two of the enzymes that break down starch into sugar
- protease and several other enzymes break down proteins into amino acids
- lipase enzymes break down the fats found in most nuts, oils, meat and dairy products into compounds called fatty acids and glycerol
- lactase breaks down a sugar called lactose that is found in milk and dairy products into its basic sugars.

These are just some of the thousands of enzymes our body makes.

If you are lacking the gene in your DNA that instructs your cells to produce a specific enzyme you are unable to digest the food to which the enzyme is targeted. The enzyme lactase is a good example of this. Without it you are lactose intolerant and unable to digest the lactose found in milk and diary products.

With the exception of identical twins, our DNA is unique to each and every one of us and the genes it contains are inherited from our parents and their parents before them. It is this inheritance that dictates not only who we are but also what enzymes we have at our disposal and hence what we can and cannot eat and digest.

Our early ancestors began farming about 10,000 years ago in a period that is often referred to as the agricultural revolution. Over the years they adapted from a hunter gatherer diet and developed the ability to digest the food that farming was making available to them. Some of this we continue to eat today. A striking example of how our DNA has changed is the ability to digest milk and dairy products. All humans are born with the ability to digest their mothers milk, but before the agricultural revolution, there were no dairy products so when children were weaned, they lost this ability. As adults they did not produce the lactase enzyme because they didn't need to. Enter the agricultural revolution and the domestication of cattle and sheep, having the ability to digest milk gave us a new protein rich food and a tremendous advantage. As a result lactose tolerance evolved in the groups of people that reared cattle but not in people like the Chinese and south east Asians who did not rear them. This ability to digest milk and diary products is still clearly seen today in ethnic groups. Figures vary but between 5% and 20% of people of Caucasian decent have a level of lactose intolerance. Around 35% of South Sea Islanders have the problem. In people of African decent the figure rises to between 65% and 70% while in some Asian populations the figure is as high as 90%.

Hormones

Hormones are part of our endocrine system. We have all heard of the hormones oestrogen and testosterone, but these are just two of the enormous number of hormones our body produces. Hormones are produced in cells in specific glands and travel to the organs that need them in our bloodstream.

Hormones are chemical substances that act as messengers. They are vital for repairing and regulating our body's functions, from simple things like feeling hungry to more complex functions like our emotions and reproduction. Some functions are easy to understand but some are extremely complex.

Unlike enzymes which are made only from amino acids, hormones are made from amino acids that are combined with other chemicals. Because of this they are classified into four groups. Steroid hormones, Eicosanoids, Amino acid derived hormones and Peptides. When it comes to 'You are what you eat' the following are the hormones are the ones we need to know something about;

- Insulin, which is produced in the pancreas, is the hormone that manages and regulates the amount of glucose that is in our blood at any one time. It helps to keep our blood sugar level from getting too high or too low and it directs surplus glucose into the liver for short term storage in the form of glycogen.
- Our thyroid gland produces a hormone called Tyroxine which among other things controls the rate at which we digest and breakdown the food we eat.
- Our adrenal glands produce Adrenaline and Cortisol which prepare our body for rapid activity, the 'flight or fight' hormone that has the effect of increasing our heart rate, increasing the amount of sugar in our blood and diverting blood to our muscles and brain.
- Leptin is made in our fat cells and this regulates our energy balance by suppressing the urge to eat. It tells us when we are full.
- Ghrelin is made in our stomach and small intestine and this tells us when to eat by making us feel hungry.

Ageing causes a drop in hormone production and a decline in our body's ability to repair and regulate itself. Because hormone production is a highly interactive process a drop in the production of one hormone is likely to have a knock on effect on the whole hormone production process, signalling to other hormone producing cells to release lower levels of hormones. As we advance in years this can potentially result in lower levels of some of the hormones we need.

Our Metabolism

The chemical reactions that transform the food we eat, the water we drink and the air we breath into the materials and compounds that make up our bodies is our metabolism. All of these chemical reactions are helped along by enzymes, usually in a sequence of steps. The more complex the food the longer the sequence of steps. The sequence of steps and the enzymes that take part at each stage of the conversion process is a metabolic pathway. Because we consume so many different types of food, each of which has a different metabolic pathway there are thousands of different metabolic pathways in our body.

Carbohydrates

Carbohydrates are the most abundant biological molecules and they fulfil numerous roles in our body. Most green plants produce carbohydrates as they use them as their energy store. The food we eat supplies us with carbohydrates in two different forms, starch and sugar. Each of these also contain fibre and cellulose. Starches and sugars provide us with energy. Fibre and cellulose provides us with the 'bulk' our digestive systems need to work efficiently.

Carbohydrates are called carbohydrates because they are made from carbon, hydrogen and water. They are organic compounds. In biochemical terms all carbohydrates, including the fibre and cellulose they contain, are sugars. Carbohydrates and sugars consist of single, double or multiple units of sugar that are joined together in different ways. Simple sugars are only one or two units long and they are typically sweet in taste whereas carbohydrates can be thousands of sugar units long. Most but not all have a starchy taste.

With the exception of a simple sugar called fructose all carbohydrates, irrespective of whether they are in the form of starchy carbohydrates or sugar, are digested and broken down in our body to form glucose, a simple form of sugar that our body uses as a source of fuel to produce energy. A series of enzymes then convert the glucose into ATP, adenosine triphosphate, the energy used by each of our cells. Simple carbohydrates and sugars require very little enzyme activity to break them down but more complex carbohydrates need to be broken down by a series of enzymes before they can be absorbed. The enzymes amylase and maltose are examples of these.

So if all carbohydrates are made from sugar and when we digest them and break them down into sugar, we need to understand what sugar is and how it is used in our body.

What exactly is sugar?

First and foremost sugar is a natural food. It only becomes unnatural when it is in a form, concentration or quantity that is not found in nature. Table sugar, extracted and refined from cane sugar or sugar beet and High Fructose Corn Syrup made from corn starch are examples of this type of unnatural sugar. Sugar comes in several forms and many disguises. The most common form is sucrose or what we know as table sugar. This is a 'dissacharide', a compound that is made up of one molecule of glucose that is linked to one molecule of fructose. So it contains 50% glucose and 50% fructose. When we eat it we break it down and convert it into separate molecules of glucose and fructose. These are both simple sugars or 'monosaccharides'. There is a third monosaccharide called galactose that is found in milk and dairy products in the form of lactose, which is one molecule of glucose and one molecule of galactose.

All other types of sugar and all carbohydrates, fibre and cellulose are made from different combinations of these three simple sugars and each of these are made from exactly the same combination of carbon and water, six atoms of carbon and six molecules of water giving them a chemical formula of $C_6H_{12}O_6$. How can something that contains the same atoms and molecules be different? Well the simple answer is that the atoms are arranged slightly differently in chains of different lengths and it is this that makes them into different sugars.

In terms of the food we eat glucose is the most important sugar as it is provides the primary source of energy that is used throughout our body. Our body stores excess glucose in our liver and muscles in the form of glycogen and this can be easily broken down back into glucose to provide energy when we need it. Galactose is the least common simple sugar and most of what we consume is converted into glucose by the liver. Fructose is mainly found in fruit but some vegetables also contain it. Fruit like apples, grapes and berries contain between 5% and 10% fructose by weight.

Unlike galactose fructose cannot be converted into glucose and then used throughout our body. If our body is desperately short of glucose our muscles can use fructose but this rarely happens with a modern diet. Our body uses fructose in a completely different way to glucose. While every cell in our body uses glucose, our liver is the only place where fructose can be metabolised in significant amounts and converted into glycogen for storage as an energy reserve. So most of the fructose we consume is converted into glycogen by the liver and if the glycogen stores in the liver are full the glycogen is rapidly converted into fat and stored in our fat cells.

Starchy Carbohydrates

Like sugar carbohydrates are natural foods and like sugar they only become unnatural when they are in a form, concentration or quantity that is not found in nature. In nature sweet and starchy things are usually seasonal and only available for a short time of the year. If you look back a long time into our evolutionary past they are quite scace nutrients so we are wired to eat a lot of them when they are available, store them as fat and use the fat to help us survive when food is scarce. Natural unrefined, unprocessed carbohydrates come with loads of fibre, cellulose, vitamins, minerals and water. The water fills you up and the fibre and cellulose slows down the rate at which the carbohydrates are absorbed in the digestive tract and converted into glucose.

Fibre and Cellulose

Carbohydrates contain two types of fibre, soluble fibre and insoluble fibre.

Insoluble fibre is a complex carbohydrate that our bodies are unable to digest. It does not dissolve in water, is not fermented by the bacteria in our digestive system and we do not possess the enzymes needed to break the links between the sugar units in the fibre apart. It provides some of the 'bulk' that our digestive system needs.

Soluble fibre does dissolve in water and it is fermented by the bacteria and micro organisms in our large intestine and then slowly broken down into simple sugars.

Cellulose is the substance that makes up most of a plant's cell walls. Just like insoluble fibre, as we do not have the enzymes needed to break the links between the sugar units apart, it passes through our systems more or less unchanged. Like insoluble fibre it provides some of the essential 'bulk' that our digestive systems need.

High Glycaemic & Resistant Starch

Starchy carbohydrates contain two types of starch. One of these is a 'high glycemic starch' that is absorbed and broken down into glucose very easily and surprisingly quickly. Because of this it gives you a fast 'sugar hit' and any glucose that is not needed as an immediate energy source is stored in the form of glycogen in various buffer stores around our body. When these buffer stores become full the excess glucose ultimately finds its way to our fat cells.

The other starchy carbohydrate is known as Resistant Starch and it is called resistant starch simply because it is much more difficult for our bodies to digest it. It takes longer to digest and the starch in it is released much more slowly, this means that it makes us feel full for longer Because it provides the benefits of both soluble and insoluble fibre some people regard resistant starch as a third type of fibre.

Insulin; how our body handles glucose

Because glucose is the essential source of energy for our body we have different ways of ensuring that the right amount of glucose is flowing in our bloodstream at any given time. Our body also makes sure that any glucose that is surplus to requirements is not wasted. Key to this is the hormone insulin. But what exactly is insulin and what does it do?

When we consume and digest carbohydrates our pancreas releases insulin. This is a hormone that,

- enables glucose to be transported across cell membranes to where it is needed as a source of energy
- when we have more glucose than we need it converts the glucose into glycogen so that it can be stored in our muscles and liver
- when the muscle and liver cells are full it helps excess glucose to be converted into fat
- because proteins and fats are important sources of food it has the effect of protecting them by preventing them from being broken down and used as a source of energy.

As glucose levels rise more insulin needs to be released, so there is a direct relationship between insulin, glucose, the carbohydrates we consume and the rate at which our body breaks down and digests the carbohydrates. The slower the rate at which the carbohydrates are converted into glucose the less insulin your body needs to produce.

Fats

Just about all natural foods contain some fat in different forms and in different amounts. Fat is in our food because like us, both plants and animals use fats as the most efficient way to store surplus energy. Meat contains animal fat, fish contains fish oil and vegetables, nuts and seeds contain vegetable oils. Commonly we hear about two types of fat, saturated fat and unsaturated fat. But what does 'saturated' mean and why is a saturated fat different to an unsaturated fat? Is one fat better than the other?

Why do we need fat?

Dietary fats are essential nutrients that are regarded as the third group of food after carbohydrates and proteins and they are the most diverse group of biochemicals in our body. Dietary fats are important:

- Every cell in our body needs fat as it forms an essential part of the membrane that surrounds the cell.
- Fats provide us with an important store of 'backup' energy. Glucose that our body does not immediately need is converted into glycogen and then into fat that is stored in fat cells. The medical term for our body fat is adipose tissue. Interestingly this fat tissue itself plays an important role in the production of some hormones that work along side insulin to help keep our blood sugar levels stable. We usually associate energy with carbohydrates but fats are actually the most energy rich food we consume. They provide us with about 9 kcal of energy per gram compared to 4 kcal energy per gram of carbohydrate or protein. This makes fat a powerful source of energy and a very efficient way of storing it.
- Our body uses fat to make vitamin D and fats also enable it to absorb and transport some of the other important vitamins it needs.
- Without fat our nerves and brain would not work properly. It forms part of the material that is wrapped around our nerve cells so it is hardly surprising that our brains contain large amounts of fat.
- Fat helps us regulate our body temperature and it also provides a protective layer around our organs.
- Dietary fats play a key role in the production of some of the essential hormones that are needed to regulate many body processes.

What are fats?

In simple terms fats are made from small chains of carbon and hydrogen atoms that are 'bound' together in small building blocks called 'fatty acids'. They are jointed together in different ways and held together at one end by a sort of 'head' that is also made from carbon and oxygen atoms. The chains come in different lengths and they are twisted together and 'bent' in different ways to make the different groups of fats. In some fats all of the available atoms of carbon and hydrogen are joined together, in others they are not and it is this that determines whether or not a fat is saturated:

- Saturated fats. A fat is 'saturated' when all of the available atoms of carbon and hydrogen are linked together and this makes saturated fats very stable. As a general rule saturated fats are solid at room temperature. The more saturated a fat is the more stable it is and the more beneficial and safer it is to eat. Saturated fats are found mostly in meat, cheese, milk, butter and eggs.
- Monounsaturated fats are the main unsaturated fats and they are liquid at room temperature. They are found in food like olive oil, avocados and peanuts.
- Polyunsaturated fats, which are often referred to as PUFA's, Polyunsaturated Fatty Acids. These are found in nuts, seeds, meat and fish, in particular cold water oily fish like salmon, herring and mackerel.

Some unsaturated fats are liquid even when they are extremely cold. In reality a food usually contains both saturated and unsaturated fat. Olive oil is a good example of this The saturated fat is dissolved in the unsaturated fat. If you put the olive oil in the fridge the saturated fat solidifies out at the bottom of the bottle leaving the unsaturated fat liquid on top.

Triglycerides, phospholipids and a group of fats called Sterols are the most commonly found members of what are called 'dietary fats'. They occur naturally and all share a common characteristic of being insoluble in water. The sterol group of fats make a wide number of different compounds that are vital to our health. In the sterol group cholesterol is a fat that most of us have heard of but the triglycerides are by far the most common as they account for 95% of the dietary fat found in our food and 99% of the fat found in our bodies.

All of the fat we consume is broken down by enzymes into its basic components of fatty acids and glycerol and it ends up inside us in the form of 'lipids', the medical term used to describe the fats that are found in our blood. These fatty acids can be used an an immediate source of energy but if we do not need the energy they are converted back into fat and stored in our fat cells.

Essential Fatty Acids or EFA's

Most of us have heard about Essential Fatty Acids, the names Omega 3 and Omega 6 usually come to mind. But what exactly are they and why are they so important?

Our bodies are able to make most of the different types of fats that it needs from the food we eat and you will be surprised to learn that cholesterol is one of them. However, some of the fats we need can only be obtained directly from our food. Because our bodies are unable to make them these fats are called Essential Fatty Acids, often referred to as EFA's. Without these essential fatty acids our body simply will not function. They fulfil numerous roles and they play a major part in supporting and maintaining our immune and cardio vascular systems.

Alpha Linolenic Acid (ALA) and Linoleic Acid (LA) are the two Essential Fatty Acid's that are of most interest as they are the 'parents' so to speak of the different groups of Omega-3 and Omega- 6 fatty acids that our bodies make from them.

- Alpha Linolenic Acid (ALA) is the parent of the Omega 3 group of Essential Fatty Acids and it needs to be converted by our body into eicosapentaenoic acid (EPA) and decosahexaenoic acid (DHA) before we can use it. Unfortunately this conversion process is not very efficient and some scientists believe that as little as 1% of the ALA we consume ends up as DHA or EPA. To make matters worse this 1% conversion process decreases even more as we get older. Luckily both DHA and EPA can be obtained directly from our food so we need to obtain a lot of DHA and EPA as well as ALA from our diet. Sadly the modern Western Diet does not provide a very good source of any of these Omega 3 fats. ALA can be obtained from both plants and animals but we can only obtain it in significant amounts and in the usable form of EPA and DHA from oily fish and marine animals.
- Linoleic Acid (LA) is the parent of the Omega 6 group of Essential Fatty Acids and it is converted by our bodies into Gamma-Linolenic acid (GLA) and Arachidonic Acid (AA).

Unlike ALA, Linoleic Acid it is readily converted into GLA and AA and our Western Diet provides an abundant source of Linoleic Acid.

In order to survive we need to eat fat and we need the right amount of the right fat in the right balance. Over the last sixty years fats have to a certain extent been demonised. We have all been led to believe that they are bad. The fat cholesterol that is found in animal products has received a particularly bad press, but cholesterol is a vital component of cell membranes and it is key to the production of some vitamins and essential steroid hormones. Because it is so important most of the cholesterol we need is made by our own cells in our liver and it is made in a carefully regulated way. Strange as it may seem, only a small amount of what we need comes from the cholesterol in the food we eat.

Vitamins

Although they are only needed in small amounts vitamins are essential for our body to function correctly. Deficiencies in any of them can cause serious health problems. Most of the compounds our body needs can be made from the nutrients in our food. Possibly because they were readily available in our food, we evolved without the ability to make vitamins so, with the exception of vitamin D, it is essential that we obtain them from our food.

The history of vitamins

Vitamins were first identified in 1905 by a British doctor named William Fletcher who was researching the causes of a tropical disease called Beriberi. In 1906 a biochemist named Frederick Gowland Hopkins discovered that certain nutritional parts of food were important to our health. It wasn't until 1911 that a Polish scientist called Cashmir Funk gave these special nutritional parts of food the name vitamine - 'vita' meaning life and 'amine' from a compound called Thiamine that he had been studying. Over the following years the vitamins as we know them today were discovered. Vitamin C is probably a vitamin we are all aware of and it has an interesting history.

For centuries scurvy was the scourge of all who sailed on long sea voyages. Thousands of sailors died each year. Everyone knew that a poor diet caused scurvy but because vitamins had yet to be discovered no one knew that a deficiency in vitamin C was the cause. After testing various foods, in 1747 a Scottish naval physician called James Lind discovered that something in citrus fruit not only prevented scurvy but also provided the quickest and most effective cure for the disease. For the Navy the problem was how to keep a supply of fresh fruit on a sailing ship that could be at sea for months on end? It was clear that food could prevent scurvy, so in 1760 the British navy supplied four ships that were setting out on long voyages with four different types of food in order to see if they would be able to prevent scurvy. Captain James Cook was one of these captains and when he set sail in the Endeavour in 1770 to observe the transit of Venus in the middle of the Pacific Ocean he was supplied with 3 tons (7860 pounds) of sauerkraut to see if it worked. Half way through the voyage when they reached New Zealand Cook had not lost a single man from scurvy and this was something that was practically unheard of in 18th century seafaring. When Cook returned to England after three years at sea, two of the crew had been treated for scurvy but not a single death was attributed to it.

Years after James Lind's discovery British sailors were given lemon or lime juice as part of their daily rations and as a result they acquired the nickname 'Limeys'. The significance of the nutritional content of citrus fruit was lost but then rediscovered by two Norwegians in 1912. Vitamin C was the first vitamin to be artificially made in 1935.

All vitamins are essential but some are more important than others. In total there are 13 vitamins and these are divided into two groups, those that dissolve in water and those that dissolve in fat. The four fat soluble vitamins, A, D, E and K are stored in our fat but the nine water soluble vitamins, the B group of vitamins and vitamin C, are not stored. They are used straight away and any that are not used are excreted. With the exception of vitamin B12 which is stored in the liver, in order to keep us in good health vitamin C and the B vitamins need to be consumed on a daily basis. A diet of fresh, natural food usually provides all of the vitamins we need. Because processing tends to destroy them many processed foods are 'fortified' with man made synthetic vitamins.

Minerals

Minerals are substances that occur naturally in non living things as well as in plants and animals. Plants take them in from soil and water. We and other animals then obtain the minerals when we eat the plants. While minerals do not contribute directly to our energy needs, they play an important part as 'regulators' of many of our body's functions.

They are essential for our bodies to work properly. Combined with various proteins calcium, magnesium and phosphate are used in the formation of our bones and some other minerals are key to some of the processes that convert the food we eat into energy.

More than fifty minerals are found in our body and about twenty-five of these are thought to be essential. Different minerals are required in different amounts and depending on how much we need on a daily basis they are classed as being 'macro minerals', 'micro minerals' or 'trace elements'. Interestingly as we progress through our life our daily requirements change. The body stores varying amounts of minerals but it needs to maintain a steady supply in order to make up for losses. Deficiencies in some minerals can have serious consequences on our health.

Water

Good old fashioned 'Adams Ale' and it is an essential part of our diet. When we have reserves of body fat we can survive for quite a long time without food but without water we die very quickly.

Our body is about 60% water and a person loses around 40 fluid ounces or just over a litre of water a day. It leaves our body in our urine, we lose it when we breath out and it evaporates from our skin. If we are in a hot climate or exercising we lose much more than 40 fluid ounces a day. So because we are losing water all the time it needs to be replaced. Many foods contain a surprising amount of water, especially some fruits and vegetables. The rest we need to obtain from pure water and other drinks.

Summary

Well these are the building blocks. The human body is complex and extremely sophisticated so it is hardly surprising that there is a lot of science going on. So if "you are what you eat" and some of the food we eat is making us ill how is it making us ill?

Chapter Two

Our Food, Our Diet & Our Health

Our diet changed, our waistlines grew and as our waistlines grew our health deteriorated. With chronic disease increasing at an alarming rate and millions dying each year from health problems that are totally preventable how is some of the food we eat making us ill?

Insulin Resistance

Glucose is the essential source of energy for our body. When we eat carbohydrates they are converted into sugar, in the form of glucose, and our pancreas quickly responds by producing insulin. Insulin's main job is to regulate the amount of glucose that is circulating in your blood and to make sure that it is available for use by your muscles and cells. Any glucose that is excess to immediate requirements is converted into glycogen so that it can be stored in cells in your muscles and liver. When the muscle and liver cells are full the insulin enables the excess glucose in the form of glycogen to be converted into fat.

The amount of insulin circulating in our bodies is directly related to both the amount of carbohydrates we consume and the 'form' in which they are consumed. Easily digested refined carbohydrates like breakfast cereals, bread and potatoes, are easily broken down and they release their sugar very quickly, but when the carbohydrates are complex they take longer to digest and release their glucose. The more carbohydrates we consume the more insulin we need to keep glucose levels properly regulated.

Over time your body becomes less and less sensitive to insulin and the amount of glucose circulating in your blood slowly creeps up. Your pancreas needs to produce more insulin in order to keep things in check. More and more excess glucose is converted into fat, you put on weight. But the story doesn't end here. In order to help us know when we need to stop eating the fat cells in our body produce a hormone called leptin. This helps us regulate our energy balance by telling us we are not hungry and do not need to eat. Because of this leptin is called the 'satiety' hormone. Strangely, the amount of leptin your body produces corresponds directly with the amount of body fat we have. When the amount of insulin circulating in our blood is high our brain becomes confused and is unable to gauge the amount of leptin we have circulating, so it assumes that we do not have enough. In other words it tells us we need to eat more, so your body ends up being locked into a sort of loop in which it wants to take in more food and consume less energy. The end result is that we eat more, put on more weight and create the need for more and more insulin. In the end your pancreas is not able to produce enough insulin to control the amount of glucose. Glucose intolerance and then insulin resistance begins to set in.

High levels of insulin in your blood correlate to glucose intolerance, insulin resistance and type 2 diabetes. Between one in three and one in four people in the west is now thought to be suffering from one of these conditions. Glucose intolerance and insulin resistance matter because you become overweight and one in three people will go on to develop type 2 diabetes within five years. When this happens, unless you change your diet, you will be facing a lifetime of medication.

Those Few Extra Pounds

Our weight, and in particular carrying too much of it, is in many cases the starting point for a cascade of ill health. Being overweight, and in particular being obese, are major factors for many chronic diseases; heart disease, stroke, kidney disease and some cancers are all linked to obesity. If you are overweight you have a higher than average risk of developing up to fifty different health problems and there are many large scale studies that reveal some sobering statistics and compelling evidence to support this.

Body Mass Index – BMI

Whether you are above or below normal weight is measured by your Body Mass Index. This is usually referred to as BMI. This index tries to relate the amount of tissue a person has in terms of muscle, bone and fat to the person's height. This provides a means of classifying people as being either underweight, of normal weight, overweight or obese. There is some debate at precisely where the dividing lines between the different classifications should be but the most commonly accepted ranges are that a BMI less than 18.5 indicates that a person is underweight, a BMI between 18.5 and 25 indicates that they are a normal weight, between 25 and 30 that they are overweight and a BMI over 30 that they are obese.

The concept of Body Mass Index was devised in the mid 1800's by a French scientist called Adolphe Quetelet who used it as part of what he called 'social physics'. The term

Body Mass Index was first used to describe the relationship between height and weight in a scientific paper written by an American nutritionist called Ancel Keys and published in 1972. In the paper he argued that BMI as a measure;

" .... if not fully satisfactory, at least as good as any other relative weight index as an indicator of relative obesity ... "

As people in the west became heavier BMI became widely used in health studies of large populations. It has been used by the World Health Organisation since the 1980's. While it is not a particularly accurate way of assessing whether an individual is over or under weight, it is now widely used as an 'indicator' as it gives a simple measure of an individuals thinness or thickness.

How too much body fat affects our health

Precisely how excess body fat affects our health is not fully understood. It used to be thought that fat tissue was just that, a means of storing surplus energy in the form of fat, but it is now apparent that body fat is much more active in terms of how our body works. The current thinking is that as well as providing us with a store of energy, fat tissue also functions as a gland that releases hormones. Some of these hormones 'get in the way' and disrupt the way our bodies produce and use insulin and when our insulin is not working properly insulin resistance can set in. One of the hormones, adiponectin, is often referred to as the fat burning hormone as it tells your body that it needs to burn fat. Strangely, the more fat you have the less adiponectin your body is able to produce, so when you are overweight or obese it becomes harder and harder to consume the reserves of fat that have built up over the years.

What is known for certain is that there are very clear links between our weight and diabetes. Around 80% of people with type 2 diabetes are either overweight or obese. But carrying around a large amount of extra weight also weakens your immune system, and as well as making you more susceptible to coughs and colds it also increases the risk that at some time in the future you will develop an autoimmune disorder.

The bottom line is that being overweight is not a good idea and being obese will most definitely cause some damage, but you don't have to be fat to get sick.

Oxidative Stress

Oxidative Stress is all about the relationship between two compounds in our bodies called free radicals and antioxidants.

Free Radicals

The majority of life forms that on earth need oxygen to live, yet one of the strange things about this is that oxygen can exist in a form that can damage living organisms by producing compounds called free radicals. These are atoms or molecules that are highly unstable because of their structure. Any molecule or atom that has a single unpaired or 'free' electron in its outer orbit is known as a free radical. Free radicals are short lived and attempt to make themselves stable by reacting with other compounds or molecules. In order to do this they either 'steal' an electron from them, bind and attach themselves to them and create a new compound or interact in various ways with other free radicals. When the compound or molecule that is attacked has its electron stolen it is 'oxidised' and it then becomes a free radical itself and so a chain reaction begins. Once the process is started it can cascade and quickly begin to run out of control.

Simply by living and deriving energy from the air we breathe and the food we eat our bodies produce free radicals. They play a dual role as they can be helpful as well as harmful. Many are needed in controlled amounts to keep us alive and in good health. Our immune system depends heavily on them. However, some free radicals can cause damage, sometimes severe damage, by reacting with and oxidising fats and proteins inside our bodies and disrupting and damaging cells.

Free radicals are all around us. We breath them in from cigarette smoke, car exhausts and air pollution, the ultra violet rays from the sun create them when we are exposed to sunlight and we consume them in our food and often in the water we drink.The existence of free radicals has been known for more than fifty years, but it is only over the last twenty to thirty years that the role they play in the development of some chronic and degenerative diseases has been discovered. An imbalance or overload of free radicals can impair our immune system and it is a potential factor in many of the modern day illnesses that are currently increasing at an alarming rate. In order for us to be able to lead healthy lives the Free Radicals need to be neutralised, rendered harmless and kept in check and to do this we need antioxidants.

Antioxidants

The word antioxidant refers to any molecule that is capable of deactivating a free radical and making it stable. Unlike free radicals which have an electron missing, antioxidants are molecules that have electrons to spare. When antioxidants come into contact with free radicals they hand over their spare electrons and neutralise the free radicals by binding to them and effectively 'making them safe'. Antioxidants are effectively scavengers and because they are designed to mop up free radicals they are stable even after they have given up their electrons.

The human body strives to keep itself in a state of balance and it has the ability to 'ramp up' its antioxidant defences when it needs to. It has a highly complex internally produced defence against free radicals, a sophisticated armoury of thousands of different types of antioxidants that is uses to defend and protect itself by inhibiting the formation of free radicals, neutralising free radicals that are already formed and repairing any damage that free radicals have caused. In addition to our bodies own antioxidant defence team, antioxidants can be obtained from the food we eat; Vitamin C, Vitamin A, Vitamin E and the beta carotenes and two groups of compounds called polyphenols and flavonoids are just some of the antioxidants that nature provides us with.

Because like us it needs to protect itself from free radicals all food, including meat, poultry, fish, eggs and plants contain antioxidants, but the amount contained in each food varies tremendously. Not all antioxidants are created equal either and they do not work in the same way. Some are expert at fighting certain types of free radicals, some dissolve in water and work in our blood and some need to be dissolved in fat to enable them to work inside our cells. Some even work as regulators that restore the antioxidant properties of vitamin C and vitamin E after they have neutralised free radicals in our body.

Oxidative Stress

Maintaining the correct balance between free radicals and antioxidants is essential for our body to work properly. A state of Oxidative Stress exists when there is an imbalance between free radicals and our body's ability to render them harmless or repair the damage they have caused. The more free radicals we are exposed to the more antioxidants our bodies need in order to keep them in check. Under normal balanced conditions free radicals are rendered harmless either by our body's own antioxidants or by the antioxidants we consume in our food. However, if we are not consuming enough antioxidants or enough of the compounds that our bodies use as 'building blocks' to make its own antioxidants, the damaging effect of the free radical remains unchecked. Our body's defenses are overwhelmed and the free radicals oxidise compounds in our body and begin to damage cells. Ultimately a state of oxidative stress sets in.

The effect of oxidative stress depends on the scale of the imbalance between the free radicals and the antioxidants. A cell is able to overcome small amounts of damage and regain its original state, but more severe oxidative stress can have toxic effects that can damage proteins, DNA and some of the fats in our bodies and, on occasion, it can result in widespread cell death that can trigger a number of chronic, inflammatory and degenerative diseases.

Metabolic Syndrome

Sometimes referred to as Syndrome X, Metabolic Syndrome is a group of conditions that are related to the way our body digests and uses food. Most recent figures suggest that 1 in 4 of the adult population in the UK and 1 in 3 of the adult population in the United States are now affected by it. However, as the prevalence of the disease increases with age, while the figures for people in their 30's and 40's would be lower, it is likely that around more than half of the over 50's in prosperous developed countries now suffer from the condition. Irrespective of what the precise figures are Metabolic Syndrome is generally regarded as having reached epidemic proportions and it is a syndrome that can creep up on us slowly without us knowing it.

While the symptoms were first observed by an Italian physician more than 200 years ago and documented by a French doctor in the late 1940's, the term Metabolic Syndrome only came into common use in the 1970's. While it is not a 'disease' as such Metabolic Syndrome is a medical term that defines a combination of risk factors that lead to the increased likelihood of developing some of the chronic illnesses that have now become so prevalent. The risk factors are;

- blood pressure that is above 'normal' levels
- high levels of blood sugar, glucose intolerance and insulin resistance
- excess body fat, in particular fat around the waist and internal organs
- above normal levels of triglycerides - one of the types of fat found in your blood

Linking all of these together is insulin. Having any one of these risk factors does not mean that you have Metabolic Syndrome but it does increase the chance that you will go on to develop cardio vascular disease. Having three or more risk factors results in a diagnosis of Metabolic Syndrome and this means the increased risk of health complications that are both long term and serious: hardening of the arteries (atherosclerosis), type 2 diabetes, heart attack, kidney disease, stroke, gout, non alcohol related fatty liver disease and cardio vascular disease are just some of them.

People suffering from Metabolic Syndrome are 5 times as likely to develop type 2 diabetes and globally, of the 400 million people with type 2 diabetes, 80% will ultimately die from cardio vascular disease. This puts Metabolic Syndrome and diabetes way ahead of HIV and AIDS in terms of morbidity and mortality and yet it is a condition that is not well recognised and rarely treated.

Our Immune System

The word inflammation comes from the Latin word *'inflammo'* meaning *'I set alight, I ignite'*. When something harmful or irritating affects a part of your body there is an automatic response to try to remove it. When you catch a cold or sprain your ankle your immune system moves into gear and triggers a chain of events that is referred to as the inflammatory cascade. The familiar signs of inflammation, raised temperature, localised heat, pain, swelling and redness, are the first signs that your immune system is being called into action and they show you that your body is trying to heal itself.

Innate & Adaptive Immunity

Inflammation is part of our body's 'innate' immune response, something that is present even before we are born. Innate immunity is an automatic immunity that is not directed towards anything specific. As we go through life and are exposed to diseases or vaccinated against them we acquire 'adaptive' immunity. In a delicate balance of give-and-take inflammation begins when 'pro-inflammatory hormones' in your body call out for your white blood cells to come and clear out an infection or repair damaged tissue. These pro-inflammatory hormones are matched by equally powerful closely related 'anti-inflammatory' compounds which move in once the threat is neutralised to begin the healing process.

Acute & Chronic Inflammation

The inflammation we experience during our daily lives can be either 'acute' or 'chronic'. Chronic inflammation is sometimes referred to as 'systemic' inflammation.

Acute inflammation that ebbs and flows as needed signifies a well balanced immune system. Colds, flu and childhood diseases mean that inflammation and a rise in temperature starts suddenly and quickly progresses to become severe. The signs and symptoms are only present for a few days and they soon subside. On occasion, in cases of severe illness, they can sometimes last for a few weeks but this is unusual. Sometimes, however, as in the case of chronic or systemic inflammation, the inflammation itself can cause further inflammation. It can become self perpetuating and sometimes last for months or even years. Symptoms of inflammation that do not go away are telling you that the switch to your immune system is stuck in the 'on' position. It is poised on high alert and is unable to shut itself off.

Chronic Inflammation & Our Health

The study of inflammation and our immune system is a relatively new science. While there is still an enormous amount to learn there is no doubt that the human immune response is an extremely sophisticated finely balanced mechanism. Without it we would not be able to survive the most minor infection or the tiniest cut. Some scientists believe that like other things in our evolutionary history, our sophisticated immune response gave our early ancestors a major survival advantage. As with so much about the human body, how such a sophisticated response came about is unclear. It is certainly the subject of a great deal of speculation. What is clear however, is that most scientists studying our immune system agree that many health conditions and chronic diseases stem from damage caused by chronic inflammation, inflammation that for some reason has run out of control.

In time we all age, some faster than others, and it is clear that when this happens our inflammatory response changes for the worse. How and why this happens is not fully understood but there is mounting evidence that ageing is associated with a chronic low level inflammation that has of late been given the name sterile inflammation. This concept goes some way to explaining why for many of us our health deteriorates and chronic diseases set in as we age.

We know from inflammatory markers and pro inflammatory and anti inflammatory hormones that in the Western World chronic or systemic inflammation is on the rise and it keeps our body in a constant state of being 'in repair' mode. While many are content to treat this inflammation with drugs, more and more medical professionals are beginning to accept that understanding and treating the underlying cause of the inflammation would be a much better long term solution.

Stress, Lifestyle & Inflammation

Does lifestyle play a part in inflammation? In a word yes, and the impact of lifestyle can be greater than you think.

Believe it or not stress can be a killer. Our body is hard wired to protect us from the threat of danger. If you have ever had a panic attack or woken from a really frightening dream in a cold sweat with your heart pounding you will understand only too well what acute stress feels like.

All human beings have a natural alarm system of '*fight or flight*' so when we are angry, anxious, tense and generally on edge our bodies produce a surge of hormones that prepare us for the fight that lies ahead. They increase our heart rate, increase our blood pressure and give rise to a sudden boost of energy. Cortisol, the primary stress hormone, increases the amount of glucose in our blood stream and it enhances the way our brain and body uses this glucose. In anticipation of any damage that is likely to occur it also alters our immune system and puts our body's inflammatory response onto high alert. The poor sleep quality and short sleep duration that comes with stress can also lead to increased levels of inflammatory markers.

The body's stress response system is usually self regulating but when stress in life is always present our body is over exposed to Cortisol and other stress hormones and these then begin to disrupt many of our body's processes, creating a state of chronic inflammation that weakens our immune system and interferes with proper glucose metabolism and the release of insulin. Ultimately this can leads to insulin resistance and a general state of oxidative stress.

Chapter Three

The Food Fibs That Changed The World

Being overweight, and in particular being obese, is a major factor in many chronic diseases. In the UK representative national surveys have measured the body mass index of the population periodically since 1980. The first survey showed that overall the majority of the population were either of normal weight or slightly underweight. Only 6% of men and 8% of women were classed as being obese. Since the first survey was undertaken obesity has increased dramatically. In 1993 between 13% of men and 16% of women were classified as being obese and by 2005 figures had risen to 23% and 25% respectively. In line with this the proportion of people of normal weight declined. These changes have occurred despite widespread media coverage, health education advice and a diet industry worth billions.

According to the Health and Social Care Information Centre more than 60% of the adult population in England is now overweight. On current estimates over half the population could be obese by the year 2050. Most people put on weight between the ages of 20 and 40 but it is clear that the problem begins in childhood. Overweight children become overweight adults.

Over the last sixty years 'average' food consumption has steadily increased in the developed countries of the world. It is thought that the amount of food each of us ate increased by as much as 20% between the 1960's and the late 1990's. On 'average' we are now consuming around 2,800 calories a day. But are calories alone the reason our weight is increasing and our health deteriorating? Could it be something to do with where the calories come from or some health hazards that are lurking inside our food.

A History of Carbohydrates & Fats

Carbohydrates and fats have been around for a long time and there is no doubt that they provide us with an essential part of our diet. But over relatively recent history the amount of carbohydrates and fat we consume, as well as the form in which they are consumed, has changed dramatically and from an historical perspective it is interesting to see why and how this happened.

Starchy Carbohydrates & Sugar

When we think of carbohydrates we immediately think of something like bread, pasta, rice or potatoes, but all vegetables, fruit, meat and diary products contain them in differing amounts. The one thing starchy carbohydrates have in common is that you can usually see them, but sugar is different. In the forms of table sugar, honey, golden syrup, maple syrup and molasses the sugar is clear to see but when it is packaged up inside other things it is invisible and this is where sugar in particular is so dangerous.

Our ancestors, the early hunter gatherers, are thought to have consumed between 50 and 100 grams of starchy carbohydrates a day and these carbohydrates would have been in a complex unrefined form with large amounts of fibre and cellulose and plenty of micro nutrients. As well as the effort involved in finding them in the first place, their bodies had to work hard to digest them and extract the glucose from them. It is estimated that the typical Western diet now contains between 350-600 grams of carbohydrate a day, an increase of between 500% and 750%, and this carbohydrate is usually highly refined and readily available. Somehow our bodies have to cope with this massive increase. Add to this the fact that our ancestors led highly active lives and today most of us lead sedentary lives and it becomes clear that we have an enormous problem on our hands.

Eating sensible amounts of complex carbohydrates is fine but eating sugar and refined carbohydrates is not a good idea. To a great extent this is all to do with how we digest and absorb the carbohydrates. The type of carbohydrate we are consuming today has a massive effect on our insulin levels simply because we are consuming highly refined carbohydrates that contain very little fibre, cellulose and resistant starch. It is these that slow down the rate at which the carbohydrates are digested, absorbed and converted into glucose and this means that we need to produce far less insulin to regulate the amount of glucose circulating in our blood. Because of this, carbohydrates high in fibre, cellulose and resistant starch create less of a 'sugar spike' in our blood. In addition to this, as your digestive tract is hard at work breaking them down you feel full for longer and as a result eat less.

Refined carbohydrates

Irrespective of where they come from all carbohydrates contain different amounts of the vitamins, minerals and antioxidants that are essential for our bodies to work properly. However, when carbohydrates are refined much, if not all of these are removed, and this makes refined carbohydrates impoverished products that have lost much of their nutritional value. In order to combat this the carbohydrates are fortified with added vitamins and minerals to replace the things that have been taken out. In the case of cereals and grains that go through a milling process chemicals are often added in order to stop the resulting powder from forming lumps. The standard white flour that we consume in a loaf of bread or a pizza is a long way from the whole grain wheat the flour came from.

The Carbohydrate Sugar

A carbohydrate we have all heard of and one that is quite rightly receiving a really bad press simply because it plays such an insidious role in our health. Man's love affair with sugar goes back a long way. For some reason we are almost wired to seek it out. But if sugar is bad for us why do we crave it? What exactly does it do to our brains that makes us want it so much?

Whenever we eat food our body produces a series of hormones. One of these is a hormone called dopamine. This is released in our brain and it plays a major role in both our motivation to eat and the reward we get from what we eat. If we eat the same thing over and over again we become bored and the dopamine levels even out. This encourages us to look for something else to eat. But when we eat sugar, no matter how much we consume, this does not happen. In people who are dependent on drugs like nicotine and alcohol the dopamine receptors are on high alert and this causes the individual to seek out the thing that gives them the 'high'. Although no where near as extreme as addictive substances, sugar causes a similar reaction in our brain. We seek it out, eat too much and give ourselves a 'sugar rush' high. The bottom line is that sugar makes us feel good.

Why this happens is interesting. It is thought to come from a time in our evolutionary past when, as a result of climate change, sugar, in the form of fruit, was only available for a short time of the year. Millions of years ago our early ancestors the apes lived in a tropical climate and were able to eat the vegetation and fruit they needed to provide them with energy throughout the year. Glucose and fructose were available from this more or less 'on demand'. As the apes moved into Eurasia, the climate cooled, the forests became deciduous and fruit was only available for a short time of the year. It became seasonal. This resulted in some very hungry apes and a species that was in decline. At some point a mutation occurred and this made some of the apes extremely efficient at processing the fructose that was found in the seasonal fruit and quickly and efficiently converting it into fat. Even small amounts could be consumed and very quickly stored as fat. This gave these apes a huge survival advantage. They ate a lot of fruit while they could, put on fat and used the fat to help them survive when food was scarce.

Today all apes, including humans, have this mutation. Our bodies have evolved to become very efficient at handling sugar, and in particular fructose, so that we can survive on very little of it. So when sugar is available we seek it out, eat too much of it and end up putting on weight.

Sugar, the first 'manufactured' food

In reality sugar is one of the first 'manufactured' foods. It was first domesticated on the island of New Guinea about 10,000 years ago. The raw sugar cane was chewed and it is thought that the juice extracted from the cane was used in religious ceremonies. Sugar spread slowly from island to island reaching mainland Asia around 1,000BC. By 500AD it had reached India where it was used as a medicine. By 600AD it had spread to Persia and when the Arab armies conquered Persia they took a love of sugar and the knowledge of how to make it back to the Middle East. As the Arab Empire grew, wherever they went sugar went with them and they more or less turned sugar refining into an industry.

Probably the first Europeans to come across sugar were the Crusaders and the first sugar began reaching Europe in small amounts. In the Middle Ages it was regarded as a spice. It was expensive and only consumed by the wealthy. Some enterprising Crusaders saw an opportunity and began farming and processing sugar cane in small amounts in Cyprus but as the Crusades came to an end the supplies from the Arabs diminished and new sources of supply were needed. The hunt was on to find places where sugar cane could be grown and it soon found its way via the Canary and Cape Verde Islands to the Caribbean.

A large amount of the sugar we consume to day is refined from sugar beet. Modern sugar beet dates back to the middle of the 18th century. The first factory for extracting sugar from beet was built in Poland in 1801. There was a rapid growth in the European sugar beet industry when the French began growing sugar beet on a large scale during the Napoleonic wars. British navel blockades had stopped the import of cane sugar so the French turned to sugar beet and improved refining techniques. By 1840 about 5% of the world's sugar came from sugar beet and by 1880 this figure had increased ten fold to 50%. The first commercial production of sugar from sugar beet began in America in 1879. With cheap imports from its far flung empire the UK did not begin growing sugar beet on a commercial scale until the mid 1920's, but as more sugar beet was planted and refined the price of sugar fell and as the price fell so consumption and demand increased. The rest, as they say, is history.

In 1700 the average Englishman consumed 4 pounds of sugar a year. By 1800 he was eating 18 pounds a year and by 1870 consumption had risen to 47 pounds. By 1900 we were consuming 100 pounds a year. Today, about 25 percent of people eating a typical 'Western Diet' consume around 95 kilograms or getting on for 200 pounds of sugar a year and for most of us this is more than our body weight. Sounds impossible? Well not when you consider that a can of 'regular' soft drink can contain up to 10 teaspoons of sugar, in other words about 40 grams. You don't drink 'regular' soft drinks? Well sugar in some form or another is added to just about all processed food because as well as enhancing its flavour it also acts as a preservative. If you look at the label carefully even tinned beans and chopped tomatoes often contain added sugar, and it is often in the form of something called High Fructose Corn Syrup.

High Fructose Corn Syrup.

When we think of sugar we immediately think of table sugar, sucrose. This is one part of the simple sugar fructose linked to one part of the simple sugar glucose. This makes it a disaccharide. As a simple sugar Fructose is found in varying amounts in fruit and some vegetables, either on its own or combined with other sugars. Contrary to what we are sometimes led to believe, sugar and fructose in particular, are not alien substances and they are not 'poisons'. When they consumed in naturally occurring amounts as part of a natural 'whole' food they are relatively benign. When vegetables and fruit are eaten as a 'whole food' and in normal amounts the nutrients, antioxidants, fibre and other compounds that they contain counter many of the detrimental effects of the sugar and fructose as the fibre slows down the rate at which the sugars are broken down and absorbed into our bodies. Any potentially adverse effects of the sugar are balanced out by the nutritional gain of antioxidants, vitamins and fibre. To put this into perspective a cup of chopped tomatoes contains 2½ grams of fructose, a medium size desert apple about 4½ grams, a 300ml can of 'regular' non diet soft drink contains around 40grams and a 'super size' can of regular soft drink has about 60 grams. From a health perspective it is strongly recommended that your daily consumption of fructose is less than 25 gram, in other words the amount in five desert apples or one 300ml can of non diet soft drink. Today it is estimated that about 10% of the calories in a typical western diet come from fructose.

So a small amount of glucose and fructose is not a bad thing. In fact, there is some evidence that a little bit of fructose on its own may help your body process glucose properly. However, consuming too much fructose, especially when it is in a pure refined form appears to overwhelm the body's ability to process it.

While table sugar is extracted and refined from cane sugar or sugar beet, High Fructose Corn Syrup is a 100% manufactured product. It does not occur naturally. As the name suggests it is made from sweetcorn, or more correctly corn starch. Just like table sugar High Fructose Corn Syrup contains glucose and fructose and the fructose in High Fructose Corn Syrup is no different to the fructose found in table sugar. Once inside your body it works in the same way irrespective of whether it comes from corn syrup, cane sugar, apples, strawberries or grapes. Only the amounts of fructose are different. Usually High Fructose Corn Syrup contains between 42% to 55% fructose, but some soft drinks are made with High Fructose Corn Syrup that contains 65% fructose and occasionally 90% fructose corn syrup is used in confectionery.

The predecessor of High Fructose Corn Syrup was cane syrup and this goes back to 1860's America, but High Fructose Corn Syrup as we know it today only became commercially available in the early 1970's after some Japanese scientists developed an enzyme that speeded up the process of extracting and converting the sugars from the cane starch. After it was declared safe by the American FDA in 1976 High Fructose Corn Syrup began to replace table sugar, particularly in soft drinks.

Almost all manufactured and packaged, processed foods now have sugar added in some form or other and High Fructose Corn Syrup provides sugar in a cheap and easy to use form. Not only is it added to food and drinks, it is also used in large quantities as a 'browning' agent in many manufactured and processed foods and this, in particular, is of great concern as people are unaware that they are consuming sugar when they eat this type of food. Something else that needs to be kept in mind is that High Fructose Corn Syrup is almost invariably made from genetically modified corn. Some people have expressed concerns about genetically modified or "GM" foods. While the jury is still out on them it could mean that in the course of time, High Fructose Corn Syrup brings with it another new set of as yet unknown dangers.

Fructose is not only just making us fat.

Unlike glucose, fructose does not directly stimulate the production of insulin, so for many years pure fructose was thought to be a good type of sugar for people with type 2 diabetes to consume.

Unlike in the sugar sucrose, there is no bond between the molecules of fructose and glucose in High Fructose Corn Syrup. Because of this when you consume High Fructose Corn Syrup the fructose and glucose is absorbed far more quickly than the fructose and glucose in table sugar. The fructose is converted into glycogen in the liver and stored so that it can be converted into glucose if the supply of glucose in your blood runs low. There is a limit to how much glycogen your body can store. The liver can store around 100 grams and our muscle tissue around 500 grams, so we can survive for around a day on our glycogen stores. If you consume a lot of fructose in the easily digested form found in soft drinks, biscuits and processed foods, the fructose simply overloads the liver's glycogen stores and it is rapidly converted into fat.

The conversion of glycogen into fat involves a process called lipogenesis and this takes place mainly in the liver. When you eat a well balanced diet this is not a particularly efficient process but if your daily consumption of fat is low and your consumption of sugar and carbohydrates is high the conversion process becomes far more efficient. The liver converts the excess glycogen into fatty acids and these are then bound together in groups of three to form triglycerides. Some of these triglycerides are stored as fat tissue and some stay in the liver and build up as fatty deposits that damage the liver and ultimately adversely affect the way it works. Over time and years of eating too much High Fructose Corn Syrup, sugar and refined carbohydrates Non Alcohol Related Fatty Liver disease can set in. Over time our weight increases and with the excess fat you can see around your middle, and the hidden fat stored inside around your internal organs, metabolic syndrome eventually kicks in.

The World Health Organisation has given guidelines that no more than 10% of your daily calories should come from sugar. For the 'average' adult this is about 50grams of sugar which is equivalent to about three tablespoons. The American Heart Association would like to see this recommendation reduced to 5% of daily calories, 25 grams of sugar.

At the present time fructose, particularly in the form of High Fructose Corn Syrup, is regarded as being the 'bad boy'. The bottom line is that unless you have a medical condition that dictates otherwise, almost without exception we do not need extra added sugar to our diet simply because all starchy carbohydrates ultimately end up as sugar in the form of glucose. So if we are eating enough carbohydrates we are getting enough sugar.

FIB 1: Saturated Fat Is Bad For You

The biggest food fib ever and it changed eating habits around the world.

Most of us have grown up believing that food high in saturated fats causes cardiovascular disease and coronary heart disease. It is a belief value that is deeply ingrained in us and it is a view supported by just about all learned bodies associated with diet, health and nutrition. But is it true?

The first association between saturated fat and heart disease was made by a Russian scientist called Nicolay Anichlov in the years just before the first world war. He fed animal fat extracted from egg yolk to rabbits and observed that the rabbits showed signs of fat deposits in their arteries. Even at the time feeding animal fat to a herbivore must have been a somewhat bizarre experiment and it is hardly surprising that the rabbits had an adverse reaction to it. Various other studies on saturated fat and heart disease went unnoticed until the 1950's.

In the 1950's heart disease was increasing at an alarming rate, especially in the United States, and the American Heart Association, together with other learned bodies around the world, decided to do something about it. President Eisenhower had suffered a near fatal heart attack in the early 1950's and this brought media attention to the problem. An eminent American nutritionist and scientist called Ancel Keys thought that there was a connection between saturated fat and heart disease. He had what is now referred to as a "lipid hypothesis". Keys had devised the American army's K rations in the second world war and undertaken a widely acclaimed study of the effects of starvation on a group of healthy men. He was highly respected and also well connected. Keys undertook a small study aimed at supporting his idea that saturated fat caused cardiovascular disease. He presented the results of the study at a World Health Organisation meeting in 1955. At the time the study was heavily criticised so Keys set out to develop a long term study that would prove that there really was a link between saturated fat and heart disease. The study was undertaken across seven countries and it has since become known as The Seven Countries Study. With World Health Organisation funding the study began in 1956 and the first results were published in 1978. The study continued for fifty years.

Ancel Keys Seven Countries Study was and still is the subject of heated scientific debate. Opinions on the soundness of the conclusions it draws are completely polarised.

Those who criticise it have gone as far as to effectively accuse Keys of tampering with the data. When he began the study Keys had preliminary data from twenty one countries but for reasons known only to himself he chose to only use data from seven of them. When the data for all twenty one countries has been analysed by other scientists a connection between saturated fat and coronary heart disease is far less clear. Despite early criticism, even before the first results were published in 1978 the general consensus among the scientific community was beginning to support Ancel Keys views. The saturated fat found in meat and dairy products was bad for us, it was making us ill. We needed to stop eating it. So based on no scientific evidence we were told to eat carbohydrates in the form of bread, cereals and potatoes instead.

The radio and newspapers caught on to the story, it made good 'news', and before long it was almost as though a war on saturated fat had been declared. But now, nearly sixty years on, we know that the advice was actually based on miss information and what ultimately turned out to be incomplete evidence. Key data on the incidence of heart disease among populations that consumed large amounts of saturated fat was omitted or simply ignored. It is interesting to note that even now, when we know that the data used was selective and flawed, many learned bodies continue to give us dire warnings about the danger of eating saturated fat.

Things got off to a slow start but by the early 1960's the campaign to stop us eating saturated fat was moving forward and gaining momentum. By the early 1970's it was in full swing. In 1977 America changed its public health advice to "*base your meals on starchy foods*" and the UK followed suit in 1983. More and more starchy foods were being consumed and more and more unsaturated fats in the form of vegetable oils, margarine and low fat spreads were appearing in the shops. We were constantly and convincingly being told that an unsaturated fat high carbohydrate diet was the healthy option. Then out of the blue in 1972 a British scientist and nutrition expert called John Yudkin sounded the alarm. It was sugar and not saturated fat that was damaging our health.

A voice in the wilderness

As early as 1957 Yudkin had voiced concerns about the danger of sugar. In the 1960's he had conducted a series of experiments on animals and humans and these showed that large amounts of sugar led to high levels of fat and insulin in the blood, risk factors he believed to be for heart disease and diabetes. He reasoned that we had been eating things like saturated fat and butter for thousands of years but up until the 1850's for most people sugar was an expensive and rare treat. Yudkin wrote;

"If only a small fraction of what we know about the effects of sugar were to be revealed in relation to any other material used as a food additive, that material would promptly be banned"

In 1972 Yudkin published his observations in a book 'Pure White and Deadly'. The book gained an international reputation but it was widely derided by some of the scientific community at the time of its publication. Yudkin's evidence relied on observations of what was happening in his experiments, but because some of the compounds and hormones involved in the process had yet to be discovered, he was unable to explain what was happening in a detailed scientific way. As a result his message was drowned out by some scientists, aided and abetted by the food industry, who were blaming the rising rates of heart disease, obesity and diabetes on the high levels of cholesterol that resulted from the consumption of too much saturated fat. A battle began between Yudkin and the *'fat is bad for you'* brigade and Yudkin's findings were ridiculed. Ultimately his reputation was ruined and the book went out of print. By the end of the 1970's John Yudkin had been so discredited that hardly anyone dared to publish anything that was negative about sugar for fear that the same thing would happen to them.

In the early 1980's scientists made discoveries that gave new credibility to John Yudkin's theories. Fructose in particular, and the way our body quickly converts it into fat vindicated his ideas. But despite mounting evidence we were still being told that saturated fat was bad. The campaign against fat was succeeding and people were eating far more refined carbohydrates and switching from saturated fats to vegetable oils. They were also eating far more low fat diet products, the label 'fat reduced' was everywhere. But instead of losing weight we gained weight, we became fatter and before we know it diabetes and chronic diseases were on the increase.

When saturated fat became the bad guy the food manufacturing industry was quick to cotton on to the fact that unsaturated fats in the form of vegetable oils and low fat foods were a massive sales and marketing opportunity. There was a problem though. When the fat was taken out the food became tasteless, so in went sugar. In the late 1970's and early 1980's sugar was expensive, but it just so happened that the move to low fat products coincided with the availability on a commercial scale of High Fructose Corn Syrup. Because of corn subsidies and improved manufacturing techniques High Fructose Corn Syrup became incredibly cheap, much cheaper than conventional sugar. As it is fairly concentrated and in a liquid form that is easy to transport, it quickly found its way into a vast number of foods. Not only did it make fat reduced food taste better, it was easy to add to the food and the food industry soon discovered that it was an excellent preservative. It extended a product's shelf life. For the food industry and the corn industry the fight against fat was a multi million dollar boon and no matter what the scientific evidence was it was here to stay. But the story doesn't end here.

Over the past few years High Fructose Corn Syrup has been gathering something of a 'bad press' and as a consequence the consumption of both High Fructose Corn Syrup and sugar is falling, albeit slowly. So where do we go from here? Well around twenty years ago the corn industry came up with another product, "crystalline fructose" and this is now being used extensively in flavoured waters, sports energy drinks and nutrition bars as well as baked goods, breakfast cereals and reduced calorie foods. It is produced by allowing fructose to crystallise out from a fructose-enriched corn syrup. This produces a product that is 98% pure fructose. In other words it contains nearly twice as much fructose as the High Fructose Corn Syrup currently being used. To make matters worse, because the absence of glucose means there is no insulin response, it is being promoted as being a 'healthier' pure fruit sugar that is good for you. Clearly, all the health problems associated with the fructose in sugar and High Fructose Corn Syrup will become even more pronounced as this product becomes more widely used.

Is saturated fat bad for us?

As a general rule the more saturated a fat is the more stable it is and the more beneficial and safer it is to eat. Because they are stable saturated fats do not oxidise and produce free radicals even when they are heated for cooking purposes.

The saturated fat and essential fatty acids found in butter, eggs, cheese and meat are foods that contain essential nutrients that provide the raw materials our bodies need to make a large number of hormones and enzymes as well as vitamin D. They also play a major part in helping to build our body's antioxidant defence team. Notwithstanding that many of us have been led to believe that saturated fats and in particular cholesterol are 'bad', in reality our bodies are desperately in need of them. They are needed to build brain and nerve tissue, they nourish our immune system, they help regulate our mood and they are one of the building blocks for many important hormones.

With the exception of people who have a gene that predisposes them to develop high levels of cholesterol, for most of us it is perfectly safe to consume saturated fats, provided they are part of a balanced diet that includes plenty of vegetables and fruit and complex carbohydrates.

For more than fifty years medical advice has been that saturated fats cause coronary heart disease. Even now we are told over and over again that this is the case. An internet search for 'saturated fat' will give you a recommended daily allowance for a man of 30 grams and for a woman 20 grams. Well you will amazed to hear that not a single study has proven that saturated fat causes heart disease. Saturated fat was given a bad press and it stuck. No one in the scientific community was prepared to put their hand up and break ranks until two large scale, systematic reviews of current literature and scientific research were published in 2014. Both studies raised questions about the link between fats and heart disease.

One, which was co-ordinated by a team at Cambridge University, was a 'meta analysis' of 72 different studies undertaken in 18 different countries with 600,000 participants. The study found that the total amount of saturated fat, irrespective of whether it was in a person's diet or measured in their blood, had no association with the risk of coronary heart disease. They also found no association between the total amount of monounsaturated fat and Essential Fatty Acids and heart disease, but they did find a significantly reduced risk of cardiovascular disease with high levels of margaric acid, a fat found in butter, milk and cheese and these are all foods that we have been told to avoid.

The second study was another large international 'meta analysis' that was peer group reviewed by the British Medical Association. The review was published on BMJOpen in July 2015. The article can be read for free if you log onto the British Medical Journal web site. The review presented a contrary position to the saturated fat is bad for you concept and concluded that,

> *"....... saturated fats are not associated with cardiovascular disease, coronary heart disease, stroke and type 2 diabetes, Trans fats are associated with all cause mortality .... dietary guidelines must carefully consider the health effects of recommendations for alternative macro nutrients to replace trans fats and saturated fats."*

However, while the BMJ peer group review was completely impartial the report itself came with a sting in the tail as four of the authors of the report have written books criticising what people refer to as the *"saturated fat and cholesterol hypothesis"* and thirteen of the authors are members of *"The International Network of Cholesterol Sceptics"*, an organisation that came into existence to challenge Ancel Keys and the scientific community's views on saturated fat. As a result, it is all too easy to claim that the report presents a biased view. However, like John Yudkin, scientific breakthroughs often only happen because of the efforts of individuals who are prepared to challenge received wisdom.

Contrary to what we have been told, saturated fats are not the "bad guys". Our bodies really do need them. They are an essential part a healthy diet and when they are replaced by other less healthy fats things can start going wrong.

Where are we now?

No doubt, because of the 'invisible' sugar in processed and low fat foods, the amount of sugar we consume has increased by more than 30% since 1990. As on average we each consume around 22 teaspoons a day, it is hardly surprising that the number of people with type 2 diabetes has nearly trebled. But we need to look at the incidence of type 2 diabetes with caution. Back in 1997 the standards for diagnosis were changed and the 'normal' range for blood sugar was lowered quite considerably. How and why this change was made is not clear but it inevitably means that with a lower threshold more people are now classed as having type 2 diabetes.

Following a YouTube video in 2009 that was viewed by more than four million people the danger of sugar has gone mainstream and John Yudkin is now seen as something of a hero. Today a vast number of diet books are focused on cutting out sugar and the foods that contain hidden sugar. Pressure groups around the world are lobbying for it to be taxed and labelled with health warnings. How the sugar, or more correctly the corn and food manufacturing industries, respond to this remains to be seen. Obesity rates in the UK are now ten times what they were when 'Pure White and Deadly' was published. Worse still, across populations levels of triglycerides are rising fast and up to one third of adult Americans are now thought to have Non Alcohol Related Fatty Liver Disease. All of this is a direct consequence of the consumption of too much sugar and over refined carbohydrates.

The legacy of the war on fat is that we are now eating more refined carbohydrates and sugar and less fat. Ironically, the so say healthy option of not eating saturated fat is one of the root causes of the obesity and ill health that is sweeping the western world. The incidence of coronary heart disease has not reduced despite major breakthroughs in medical treatment. Around four hundred million men, women and children around the world have been conned into adopting an untested and scientifically unproven high carbohydrate low fat diet that is having disastrous consequences.

This one big fib, that saturated fat is bad for you, led to a cascade of fibs and misinformation about food that have changed eating habits around the world.

FIB 2: Polyunsaturated Vegetable Oils Are The "Heart Healthy" Option

How the world's scientists and nutritionists got refined carbohydrates and sugar so wrong for so long is an interesting question, but the war on saturated fat brought with it yet more dangers to our health. We were told to eat more unsaturated fat in the form of Polyunsaturated Vegetables Oils because they were the healthy option. This is the second big fib about food.

If you asked the question which is worse for your health, white flour, sugar or polyunsaturated vegetable oils, most people would answer white flour or sugar. But are they really as bad as they are made out to be? They have both been around for quite a while. Just look at some Victorian and Edwardian cookbooks. People ate them then and they were generally far healthier than we are today. In reality white flour and sugar are not fundamentally bad. What is bad is the utterly enormous amounts of them that we are now consuming on a daily basis. On the other hand polyunsaturated vegetable oils as we know them today are something that did not exist a hundred and fifty years ago. They are new, entirely unnatural foods and because of the damage they can cause, they are being described by some as the 'health villains' of the 20th Century.

The story of polyunsaturated fats & oils

People have been extracting oil from nuts and seeds for thousands of years. We know that olive oil goes back to at least 3000BC and there is plenty of archaeological evidence of poppy seeds, sesame seeds, cotton seeds, linseed and almonds being processed into oil as long ago as the bronze age. However, the extraction processes used then were time consuming, not very efficient and only small amounts of oil were produced. As a consequence these oils contributed only a small amount to people's diets. A step change in the large scale production of vegetable oils came in the 1850's when solvents were first used as part of the extraction process, but even then the oils were only produced in relatively small amounts and they remained precious commodities. Over time as solvent extraction and purification techniques became more efficient vegetable oils became widely available and prices dropped. Soy bean oil became widely available in 1950's America and corn oil followed in the 1960's. When canola oil, a genetically modified rapeseed oil, was developed by the Canadians in the mid 1970's the vegetable oils as we know them were becoming well established in the market place. Today we have an enormous range of different nut and seed oils available to us.

The problem with vegetable oils

Even in their natural state polyunsaturated fats and oils oxidise and produce free radicals very easily and this is why nature has packaged them up inside nuts and seeds that are packed full of the antioxidants and vitamins needed to protect them from being oxidised. As a consequence, once the oils are extracted from the nuts and seeds at high temperature and high pressure these oils become chemically highly reactive and are characterised by very high levels of free radicals.

Polyunsaturated fats are found in different amounts in all natural foods including meat, fish, vegetables and seeds. In general, vegetable oils such as sunflower, safflower, corn, soy and canola oils are the most concentrated sources of polyunsaturated vegetable oils in our diet. The problem with all of these is the amount of free radicals they contain and the load that these put on our body's antioxidant defences. Consumption of such chemically altered oils disrupts our normal metabolism. The richer the oil in polyunsaturated fatty acids and the longer it is exposed to heat, light and oxygen, the lower the quality of the oil becomes, the more free radicals it contains and the more damage it is capable of causing.

Because the flavour of poor quality highly oxidised oils can be masked by heavy seasoning, the lowest quality oils are often used in the manufacture of salad dressings and mayonnaise. Ironically these are often presented as being the 'healthy' low fat option. Even the premium priced cold-processed oils sold in health food stores, can also contain damaging free radicals because as soon as the oil is extracted and exposed to oxygen and light it begins to oxidise. Irrespective of whether they are cold pressed or heat extracted, heating any type of polyunsaturated vegetable oil to high temperatures to fry food will compound the problem. When any oil is heated, the rate of oxidation increases at an alarming rate, doubling with every ten degrees centigrade rise in temperature, so the more the oil is heated the more free radicals are produced.

Today each of us is consuming on average around 35Kg of vegetable oil a year. It has been estimated that in a typical Western diet around 30% of a days calories come from polyunsaturated oils in one form or another. This is an astonishingly high figure and research indicates that this amount is far too high. The best evidence suggests that the daily intake of polyunsaturated vegetable oils should be around 4% of our calories. No one ever ate oils like this a hundred and fifty years ago because they simply did not exist. Where do the vegetable oils we get come from? Salad dressings, mayonnaise, fried foods, chips, fries, cakes, biscuits and processed foods. Its a long list and more often than not we are eating them without even realising it.

Why are polyunsaturated vegetable oils bad for us?

Put simply our bodies are unable to handle them, especially in the amounts we are currently consuming them in. Our bodies need polyunsaturated vegetable oils but only in very small amounts. For almost all human history vegetable oils have been consumed only as they occur naturally in nuts and seeds, and nuts and seeds are complex foods that contain many other nutrients as well as the polyunsaturated vegetable oils. It is only since industrialised extraction processes came onto the scene that we have consumed these oils in large amounts.

In all mammals cell tissues are made up mainly of saturated and monounsaturated fats. Polyunsaturated fats like the essential fatty acids Omega 3 and Omega 6 are only needed in relatively small amounts. What makes polyunsaturated vegetable oils so bad for us is the large amount of them we now consume and the residual amount that we have left in our bodies.

Polyunsaturated vegetable oils are essentially unstable and easily affected by things around them. They come complete with their own supply of free radicals plus the free radicals that they have inherited from the manufacturing process. However, once they are inside our body the polyunsaturated vegetable oils undergo a further process of oxidation and this results in yet more free radicals. The oxidised fatty acids that result from this have the potential to create an enormous amount of damage to our cells and blood vessels as well as to the DNA inside our cells. When we consume polyunsaturated vegetable oils in large amounts they are increasingly incorporated into cell membranes and because they are unstable the cell then becomes fragile. This leads to cells being damaged and the damaged cells produce more free radicals. As a consequence, these oils put an ever increasing load on our body's need for antioxidants. When our diet is lacking in antioxidants and the essential minerals and trace elements that are needed to make our internally produced antioxidants the balance tips in favour of the free radicals and a state of oxidative stress begins to develop. But the storey doesn't end here. In the course of time more and more damaged cells leads to chronic inflammation and this inflammation is 'fuelled' by the polyunsaturated vegetable oils.

Chronic & systemic inflammation

Inflammation is a bit like an iceberg floating in the ocean. The top, like the visible signs of inflammation, is clear to see, but under the surface there is an awful lot of ice, completely hidden from view. Chronic and systemic inflammation is like the ice below the surface. There are some chemical markers inside our bodies and these indicate how inflamed our bodies are. By measuring these markers across large populations it is clear that those of us who consume a typical western diet that is high in polyunsaturated vegetable oils have high levels of inflammatory markers.

Polyunsaturated vegetable oils contain different types of fats. These are broadly classified into four groups; Omega 3, Omega 6, Omega 9 and conjugated fatty acids. As well as playing several crucial roles in our body the Omega 3 group of essential fatty acids, EPA and DHA, and the Omega 6 essential fatty acids, GLA and AA, play a key role in our immune system.

Without getting into too much detail, there is a complicated interaction between the hormones and chemical messengers that form part of our immune system; cytokines, prostaglandins and some short lived hormones inside our cells called eicosanoids. Understanding a little about the eicosanoids is key to understanding the role polyunsaturated vegetable oils play in chronic inflammation. Eicosanoids can act as both pro-inflammatory compounds that 'fuel' inflammation and anti-inflammatory compounds that can calm it down by putting a sort of brake on when an immune response is no longer needed. Eicosanoids are derived from the Omega 3 and Omega 6 essential fatty acids. The Eicosanoids derived from Omega 3 are anti inflammatory and the Eicosanoids derived from Omega 6 are pro inflammatory. In order to maintain a healthy inflammatory response we need both of these eicosanoids in a relative state of balance. However with high levels of Omega 6 essential fatty acids and low levels of Omega 3 essential fatty acids we end up making far too many pro-inflammatory eicosanoids and not enough of the anti-inflammatory ones.

All commercially available vegetable oils contain large amounts of Omega 6. Safflower oil is the worst offender with a massive 75% Omega 6 and like sunflower oil, corn oil, cotton seed oil, sesame oil and peanut oil it contains no Omega 3. Only soy bean oil, canola oil, walnut oil and flaxseed oil contain Omega 3 and, with the exception of flax seed and Canola oil, the ratio of Omega 6 to Omega 3 is not good in any of them. Soy bean oil is 51% Omega 6 and 7% Omega 3 and walnut oil is 52% Omega 6 and 10% Omega 3. Canola oil, a rape seed that has been 'engineered' to have a better ratio, is 20% Omega 6 and 9% Omega 3 but because it also contains high levels of monounsaturated fats it falls into a "not quite so bad" category. With 14% Omega 6 and 57% Omega 3 flax seed oil is the only 'healthy' vegetable oil. What about olive oil? Well, it contains 75% monounsaturated fats, 13% saturated fats and 12% polyunsaturated fats of which 10% are Omega 6 and 2% Omega 3. As it is also rich in compounds that have antioxidant and anti-inflammatory properties olive oil is a very healthy oil and it is an oil that has stood the test of time.

In the good old days when Omega 3 and Omega 6 fats were obtained naturally from food that was unprocessed things were quite well balanced. We were consuming them in the ratio of one Omega 3 to one or two Omega 6. With the advent of polyunsaturated vegetable oils this ratio changed dramatically and it changed over an astonishingly short period of three or four decades.

Our diet today provides an abundant source of the Omega 6 fatty acids in the form of vegetable oils, margarines, fries, chips, snacks, fried food, processed food and baked goods, but an extremely meagre source of Omega 3 fatty acids. The only significant and easily assimilated source of Omega 3 oils comes from oily cold water fish and sadly fish like this, that is not covered in batter and deep fried in vegetable oil, features on only a few people's menu. Figures vary, but it is thought that many of us are now consuming twenty times more Omega 6 oils than Omega 3 and worse estimates are that this figure could be as high as fifty times more Omega 6 than Omega 3. This imbalance creates a highly inflammatory environment that has a profound effect on our health. Many scientists believe that this Omega 3 to Omega 6 imbalance is the primary reason for what they see as an epidemic of heart disease, high blood pressure, diabetes, obesity and degenerative diseases. Put simply, polyunsaturated vegetable oils are taking their toll. Add to this the increased load of free radicals that the polyunsaturated vegetable oils bring with them and it is easy to see that our body and our immune system is being put under enormous stress.

FIB 3: Margarine Is Healthier Than Butter

Is Margarine a healthier option than butter? Well for years we have been told that it is. However, a process called 'hydrogenation' is used to convert polyunsaturated fats that are liquid at room temperature into trans fats that are solid at room temperature. In reality trans fats are Polyunsaturated Vegetable Oils in their worst possible form and they are found in just about all of the processed food we eat. Margarine is a healthier option than butter is the third big fib about food.

A history of margarine and low fat spreads

Margarine was invented in France in 1869 during the Franco Prussian wars. It was designed to provide the army and the lower classes with a cheap substitute for butter. It was originally made from beef fat but in America, by the late 1800's, cotton seed and soy bean oils were being added to the beef fat in order to reduce costs.

In the late 1890's a process called hydrogenation was developed and this changed the structure of vegetable oils and makes them solid at room temperature. The process was further developed by a German chemist and he patented the process in 1902. By the early 1900's, with further advances in industrial processes, more vegetable oils were being used. They were a cheaper option and gradually they completely replaced beef fat. By 1945 and the end of World War 2 almost all margarine was being made from hydrogenated vegetable oils. The margarine industry was growing fast and by the late 1970's and early 1980's milk, cream and dyes were being added to create the margarine and low fat 'spreads' we know today.

The process of hydrogenation

The manufacturing process of Hydrogenation is far from being a healthy process and not surprisingly the end result of the process is not a healthy product. Polyunsaturated oils that are already heavy in free radicals are mixed with a catalyst that is then subjected to hydrogen gas in a high pressure, high temperature reactor. Hence 'hydrogenated'. Emulsifiers and starch are then added to improve the consistency and the oil is again subjected to high temperatures in order to steam clean it and remove any unpleasant smells. Bleach, dyes and flavours are then added to make it look like and taste like butter. By the time margarine reaches your table it is a completely unnatural product and hardly the healthy food it is promoted as being. Trans fats are polyunsaturated vegetable oils in their worst possible form.

So what is the problem with margarine and these low fat spreads? Well it is all to do with the trans fats. Trans fats are unsaturated fatty acids that have had their structure changed. They occur in small amounts in nature but in very large amounts in margarine and low fat spreads and over the years they have been consistently shown to be associated with coronary heart disease. Because the trans fats mimic naturally occurring fats the body doesn't recognise them as being different and as a consequence they are not excreted. Instead, just like any other naturally occurring polyunsaturated fat they are incorporated into cell membranes where they wreak havoc, disrupting the cells metabolism. In the process free radicals are produced. The end result is inflammation, yet more free radicals and more pressure on our body's antioxidant defences.

Full and partial hydrogenation

You have probably seen *"hydrogenated vegetable oils"* and *"partially hydrogenated vegetable oils"* on food labels. Trans fats are produced when vegetable oils go through a partial hydrogenation process. When oils are fully hydrogenated trans fats are not produced. Current thinking is that fully hydrogenated oils are not as bad for us as partially hydrogenated ones, but more work is needed before we can fully understand the effect they have on our health.

Fully and partially hydrogenated vegetable oils are very different. When liquid vegetable oils are fully hydrogenated they become completely solid at room temperature and this makes them more stable when they are on the supermarket shelf. When the oils are partially hydrogenated the resulting fats are semi solid at room temperature. The problem with the partially hydrogenated fats is that they contain the trans fats that are known to have harmful effects. In contrast fully hydrogenated oils effectively become saturated fats and as they contain no trans fats they are thought to have no significant effect on our health.

Fully hydrogenated oils are now being used as a supposedly healthy replacement for partially hydrogenated oils. Food manufacturing companies often blend fully hydrogenated oils with liquid oils and put them through a process called interesterification. This is a process that has been around for about twenty years. It was initially developed to produce cooking oils that oxidised more slowly than conventional polyunsaturated vegetable oils. By industrially modifying their structure and adding synthetic antioxidants these oils were made more suitable for deep fat frying. The process of interesterification changes the structure of the oil so that even though it does not contain any trans fats it performs like a partially hydrogenated oil. Sounds great, but we do not yet know whether fats that have gone through an interesterification process bring with them their own adverse health consequences.

Where are we now

A strong correlation between hydrogenated fats and heart disease was observed as long ago as the late 1940's, not long after margarine became widely available. By 1956 suggestions began appearing in scientific literature that trans fats could be the cause of the increase in coronary heart disease. Remember, this was about the time we were being told that saturated fat was to blame. For three decades these concerns were not widely addressed. To a certain extent they were hushed up. By the 1980's the war on fat was in full swing and we and the fast food companies were being urged to switch to margarine and low fat spreads. Studies in the 1990's brought renewed scrutiny on trans fats and this confirmed the negative impact they were having on our health. In 1994 it was estimated that they were causing the death of 20,000 Americans each year from heart disease. Labelling legislation was introduced in several countries and activists began campaigning to change the practices of food manufacturing companies.

In 2013 the Federal Drug Authority in America issued a determination that partially hydrogenated vegetable oils which contained trans fats were not "*generally recognised as safe*" and this was expected to lead to a ban on the use of industrially produced trans fats in American food. On 16 June 2015 the FDA finalised this determination that they were not generally recognised as being safe and set a three year time limit for their removal from all processed foods. Why this took more than seventy years, during which time they were being widely promoted as being the healthy option, is a question that will probably never be answered.

The damage to our health has been done. So what replaces trans fats? Believe it or not saturated fat in the form of lard or palm oil. While lard is a by product of the production of pork meat, increasing the amount of palm oil that is used raises some enormous environmental questions. The other options are to use 'fully' as opposed to 'partially' hydrogenated vegetable oils or 'interesterified fats'.

Trans Fats in the form of margarine and shortening have the commercially pleasing property of being able to extend a products shelf life. They are also cheap. As a consequence they are widely used in manufactured and processed foods. Look on a label and you will see 'hydrogenated vegetable fat' as one of the ingredients. Margarine, vegetable shortening, non dairy creamers and non dairy whipped toppings all contain trans fats, as do most of the biscuits, cakes and 'junk' food in your local supermarket.

For years margarine and low fat spreads have been presented as the healthy option but instead of improving our health they leave behind them the legacy of a generation of people whose health has been damaged by them. As with the polyunsaturated oils from which they are derived, no one ever ate food like this years ago because it simply did not exist.

Trans fats, partially hydrogenated and fully hydrogenated vegetable oils are a minefield. What can you do about it? Read the ingredients list on the label. If you see "partially hydrogenated vegetable oil" it means that some trans fat is present. Even if the label says zero trans fat it does not mean that the product is free from trans fat as an amount less than half a gram per serving, a serving usually being one teaspoon, does not have to be declared in most countries. Some products contain both partially and fully hydrogenated oils. So if the label says "hydrogenated vegetable oil" you do not know if it is fully or partially hydrogenated and, with current legislation, the label will not tell you whether or not the oil has been interesterified. When it comes to eating margarine the best advice is to give it a miss and eat butter instead.

FIB 4: Fruit Juice Is A Healthy Way To Start The Day

When it comes to sugar we are being well and truly 'conned' into thinking that certain foods are healthy when they are not. Fruit juice is widely promoted as being one of your five a day and a healthy way to start your day. Not true. Fruit juice is the fourth big fib about food.

Several generations of us have grown up believing that fruit juice is good for us; it boosts our immune system, helps us fight off colds, it provides us with a healthy dose of vitamin C and it counts as one of our "five a day" portions of fruit and vegetables. Have you even wondered where "five a day" came from or whether there is any scientific basis for it? Well "five a day" depends on where you live. In the UK it is "five a day" but in the United States is it "nine a day", in Australia it is "seven a day, five vegetables and two fruit" and in many European countries it is "six a day".

In 1991 a partnership programme was formed between America's National Cancer Institute and an organisation called The Produce for Better Health Information. its purpose was to persuade the American population to eat more fruit and vegetables. It was a highly successful marketing campaign but at the time there was no scientific research to back it up. Ironically it was a marketing campaign that actually did have the potential to improve our health. We now know that eating a diet rich in vegetables and fruit will reduce the risk of developing many types of cancer, high blood pressure, heart disease, stroke and diabetes. The World Health Organisation are now advising us to eat at least five and up to nine portions of vegetables and fruit a day. Sadly most of us believe that fruit juice first thing in the morning is one of them. Despite some recent adverse publicity about fruit juice, the market research company Mintel found that in the UK 76% of the people surveyed still believe this to be true, fruit juice is a healthy way start to the day. Why we believe this is an interesting story that goes back to 1920's America.

Around this time, when we were first beginning to learn about vitamins, 'acidosis' was the big health scare as it was thought to be the root of all evil. All of our ailments were linked to it. An eminent nutritionist called Elmer McCollum blamed 'acidosis' on a diet rich in bread and meat and part of his solution to the problem was to eat citrus fruit and drink fruit juice. Was he right?

Well acidosis or '*your blood is too acidic*' is something we often hear today and while it is not a food fib as such, it is a topic that is shrouded in misinformation. So where does acidosis fits into the big picture?

Acidic food and acidosis

Acidity and alkalinity are measured by pH, which stands for the Power of Hydrogen. On a scale of 0 to 14, the lower the pH the more acidic a solution is and the higher the pH the more alkaline the solution is. When a solution is neither acid or alkaline it has a pH of 7 which is neutral. Pure water is generally considered to have a neutral pH of 7. Water is the most abundant compound is our body. In fact about 60% of our body is water. Our body has an acid to alkaline ratio of between 7.35 and 7.45, so it is slightly more alkaline than pure water. If the pH of your blood falls below 7.35 the result is the condition called acidosis. If it rises above 7.45 the result is alkalosis. The pH of our blood is tightly regulated by a complex system of buffers that are continuously at work striving on a moment to moment basis to balance our pH and keep it in the range 7.35 to 7.45. When this balance is severely compromised medical problems occur, you are ill.

So is it true that the food and drink we consume causes our blood to become more acidic or more alkaline?

Well contrary to what they thought then and what we are sometimes led to believe now, the answer is "well sort of". As part of simply living our cells are continuously producing energy and in the process of doing this a number of different acids are formed and released into our body fluids. When we consume food and drink the end products of digestion and the assimilation of nutrients often results in the food having an acid or alkaline forming effect. Fortunately our body has three major buffer mechanisms that work constantly to prevent dietary, metabolic and other factors from pushing the pH of our blood outside of the 7.35 to 7.45 range. When people encourage you to '*alkalise your blood*' most of them mean that you should eat plenty of foods that have an overall alkaline forming effect.

Under normal circumstances this works fine but if you spend years eating a diet that is highly acidic these buffers ultimately become exhausted and the body has to call on its reserves, in particular its reserves of a compound called calcium phosphate. When this happens it heads in the direction of our bones, our joints and our teeth and it takes small amounts of calcium phosphate from them. Ultimately over time this can lead to some undesirable changes in your health and the onset of chronic inflammation.

So which foods have an alkaline forming effect and which have an acid forming effect? Well most wheat, grains, animal products, sugar, alcohol and highly processed foods have an acid forming effect and generally speaking most vegetables, fruit and natural unprocessed foods have an alkaline forming effect. Compared to vegetarians, people who eat large amounts of animal protein, particularly in the form of meat, lose between two and four times the amount of calcium from their calcium phosphate reserves. The larger the amount of animal protein, over refined and processed foods consumed the greater the loss of calcium. Unfortunately vegetables, fruit and unprocessed foods are in short supply in the typical western diet both now and back in the 1930's. Notwithstanding that clinical acidosis and alkalosis are medical conditions, to a certain extent Elmer McCollum was right in so far as his believed that eating too much meat and refined flour was putting pressure on our pH buffer systems, but eating citrus fruit and drinking fruit juice alone were not going to resolve the problem.

The history of fruit juice

In the late 1920' at the time Elmer McCollum was writing about acidosis, orange juice was not very popular. It was usually canned and the canning process gave it a sterilised and unpleasant metallic taste. With the suggestion that fruit juice would provide a cure the orange growers of Florida leapt on the acidosis band wagon and used it promote their products. As a result sales of orange juice increased.

With the coming of World War 2 American fruit growers got another boost when the government were looking for a way of providing the troops overseas with a supply of vitamin C. They invested heavily in research and, although it was too late for the war, by 1947 scientists had developed a way to remove water from fruit juice, freeze the concentrate for long term storage and then add water back in and convert it into a palatable drink. Sales of fruit juice exploded. By 1949 the state of Florida was producing ten million gallons of concentrated orange juice a year. Consumers quickly latched on to the idea of concentrated canned orange juice that was cheap, convenient and of course packed with vitamin C, something we all needed. All you had to do to prepare the juice was thaw it out, add water and give it a stir.

While the research in America was going on war time Britain was at the height of rationing and babies and young children were being given rose hip syrup, black current juice and concentrated orange juice as a health supplement. As this continued well into the 1950's it is hardly surprising that this gave rise to a generation in the UK that believed that fruit juice was good for you.

By the 1980's food technologists had developed a ready to serve fruit juice that tasted fresher than the frozen juice. Drinking orange juice and fruit juice was marketed not just as being 'healthy' but also as a stylish and modern thing to do. By the 1990's the first 'not from concentrate' juices were developed and marketed as 'fresh' juices packaged in very convenient cartons that could be stored at ambient temperature.

Fruit juice, and in particular orange juice, are now commodity products that are traded on the futures market. In fact they have a history of futures contracts going as far back as 1966. However, global demand has fallen slowly over the last ten years. Orange juice in particular has seen a worldwide market fall from 2.5 million tonnes in 2008 to just under 1.8 million tonnes in 2015. Whether this is the result of some justly deserved bad press or increasing interest in the Atkins and Paleo diets which do not allow fruit juice remains to be seen.

Where will the industry go from here? Well read food labels carefully because *'no added refined sugar'* is something we are seeing more and more and it usually means that concentrated fruit juice is being added instead as a sweetener.

The manufacture of fruit juice

As 'chilled' fruit juice that is made from freshly squeezed juice has a shelf life of only around twelve days, it is easy to see why so much of the fruit juice we consume is made from concentrate. As a general rule the more processed a food is the more potential there is for nutrients to be lost and this holds true for fruit juice. As an example orange juice made from concentrate has 20% less vitamin C and half the beta carotene of freshly squeezed juice.

As well as increasing shelf life concentrating fruit juice significantly reduces the cost of transportation. During the concentration process most of the water is removed from the juice. At the end of the process the fruit juice is about 65% sugar by weight. Extraction usually involves the addition of chemicals, filtration and then evaporation which involves heating the juice to high temperatures. The heat of course destroys the vitamin C. As a consequence fruit juice made from concentrate contains added vitamin C in the from of citric acid or ascorbic acid. As flavour and aroma are both lost during the evaporation, concentration and storage process something called ethyl butyrate is added to give the juice a natural aroma that people associate with freshness. Freshly squeezed orange juice contains about 1.19 milligrams of this a litre whereas juice made from concentrates contains levels as high as 8 milligrams a litre.

We all know that labels can be deceiving and we all know that fruit and citrus crops are seasonal. Even when the label on a carton of fruit juice says 'not made from concentrate' does it actually mean that the fruit juice is 'fresh'? More often than not the fruit juice has been extracted and then stored in large storage tanks in an oxygen free atmosphere. As the flavour of the juice suffers during storage flavouring is added before the fruit juice is put into cartons, but as this flavouring is made from essence and oils extracted from the fruit at the beginning of the process they do not have to be listed as an ingredient.

Why is fruit juice bad for us?

At the present time fruit juice, in a modest recommended serving of 150ml, counts as one of your 'five a day' foods but there is mounting pressure to have it 'de listed'. Notwithstanding that the processing of fruit juices strips away a lot of its nutritional value, lack of fibre and too much sugar are the key problems. When we eat whole fruit the fibre in the fruit slows down the rate at which the sugar in the fruit is absorbed and as it makes its way slowly through our digestive tract it also makes us feel full. Without the fibre the sugar in fruit juice is absorbed more or less immediately, very much like the sugar in a can of regular soft drink.

If you asked the question which contains most sugar, a can of coca cola or a glass of apple juice most people would say coke and they are correct, but only just. The sad fact is that a 350ml can of regular coke contains 40g of sugar, about 10 teaspoons and a 350ml glass of apple juice contains 39g, one gramme less and just under 10 teaspoons. If you look at it another way a 250ml glass of fruit juice has more sugar than the average size bowl of sugary breakfast cereal.

So what about the fibre. A 100 gram portion of a whole orange contains on average 1½ grams of fibre and 6.4 grams of sugar. A 100 gram portion of orange juice however contains no fibre and 10 grams of sugar. Doesn't sound too bad? Well it does when you consider that the average orange weighs about 150 grams and, despite a recommended serving of 150ml, the average glass of fruit juice is 300ml or around 300 grams. The whole orange provides 2.2 grams of fibre and 9.6 grams of sugar that is released slowly while the orange juice provides no fibre and 30 grams of sugar which is absorbed more or less instantly. In other words 3 times as much sugar and the sugar is in your bloodstream within minutes. With current maximum guidelines of 35g of sugar a day for a man and 25g of sugar a day for a woman the scale of the problem becomes clear.

FIB 5: Use Artificial Sweeteners Instead Of Sugar

No, because they are bad for you and strange as it may seem they make you fat. This is the fifth big fib about food.

Going 'sugar free' is not easy. Most of us like the taste of sugar and the sugar high and feeling of well being that it gives us. So should we retrain our palette and not eat sugar at all or change from sugar to artificial sweeteners?

Over the years scientists and food technologists have developed many different types of artificial sweeteners. Like sugar these taste sweet but they provide fewer calories. While they may satisfy our cravings for sweet things there is a lot of controversy over whether they are good for us and whether they actually damage our health.

Today the four main artificial sweeteners on the market are;

- Sucralose, the sweetener found in Splenda.
- Aspartame which is sold under the name of Equal and Nutrasweet and found in many 'diet' drinks.
- Saccharin, which because of a health scare many years ago is not often found these days.
- Stevia, a relatively new kid on the block which is sold under various brand names

With the exception of Stevia, all of these artificial sweeteners are man made products that are not found in nature and they are all known to have side effects. Most have been linked to various levels of toxicity. Aspartame continues to be the subject of great debate and despite many studies a large question mark still hangs over it.

Without getting in to the detail of the different types of artificial sweeteners, their various side effects and alleged toxicity, the main reason to avoid them is all about their purpose. At the end of the day artificial sweeteners are about reducing the amount of sugar we consume. But all the evidence shows that in the long term they actually increase our daily intake of food and calories. Put in very simple terms artificial sweeteners confuse our brain in terms of the hormones it produces when we eat. Because our body does not get the sweet things it is expecting, it feels cheated, it doesn't get the 'sugar kick', the glucose 'high'. The end result is that we end up eating more. Over time the end result is that we end up eating more of the wrong things because artificial sweeteners also influence our taste in food. We begin craving more and more carbohydrates and more and more sugary sweet things.

Artificial sweeteners also influence our eating habits in other ways. When we consume food and drink that contains them we are less likely to make healthy choices with regard to the other food we eat. Because we feel that we have in some way restrained ourselves and done the 'right thing' by not consuming sugar, indulging ourselves a little in the other food we eat is a fairly natural response. More often than not the result of this indulgence are some unhealthy choices that end up in us consuming more calories than we would otherwise have consumed.

There is plenty of evidence out there that tells us that artificial sweeteners are not a good idea. Their use consistently leads to increased calorie intake and not reduced calorie intake. It is an undisputed fact that the weight and Body Mass Index of people who consume low calorie 'diet' drinks on a regular basis is consistently higher than the BMI of people who do not drink regular or diet drinks. But consuming more calories and making bad food choices is not the only reason why this happens. Strange as it may seem, artificial sweeteners appear to favour the growth of certain types of bacteria in our digestive tract. These bacteria somehow have the ability to extract extra energy from food, so from a given meal they make more calories available to us. Ultimately these extra calories end up as fat and lead to a higher Body Mass Index.

Are Cholesterol, Statins & Plant Sterols Fibs In Waiting?

"Statins prevent 80,000 strokes and heart attacks each year in the UK, study finds"

"A third of adults should take Statins new research suggests"

We have all read the headlines. Are they fact or are they fiction?

In the 1950's saturated fat was the demon and Ancel Keys "lipid hypothesis" and the war against saturated fat has severely damaged our health. We are now faced with another demon, cholesterol. For some reason we, the media and the medical profession are currently obsessed with cholesterol levels and the need to use drugs to reduce them. At this point in time there is plenty of miss information about cholesterol and very few facts. As a result it is easy to become very confused. What we are now being told about cholesterol and the cholesterol lowering drugs we are being encouraged to take could, in the course of time, become another fib. While they may not make us fat, are what the media refer to as 'cholesterol busting' drugs and 'heart healthy' plant sterols another ticking bomb in terms of our health? Is cholesterol bad for us? Should we be taking Statins and eating margarine that contains plant sterols?

What is cholesterol

Cholesterol is one of the saturated fats that is found in animal products. It is a fat that has and still is having a particularly bad press. Unlike other saturated fats cholesterol is essential for human life. Without cholesterol we die. It is a vital component of cell membranes and our nerves, our body needs it to make vitamin D and it is key to the production of some essential steroid hormones like our sex hormones and Cortisol, the 'fight or flight' hormone that enables us to respond to stress. Cortisol is also one of the many hormones that regulate our metabolism. Even though it is only around 2% of our body weight our brain contains 25% of our body's cholesterol. Our brain, nerves and whole nervous system effectively runs on cholesterol.

Because cholesterol is so important to us our body makes it. With the exception of red blood cells, every cell in our body is able to do this. Most cholesterol however, is made in our liver from fats, proteins and sugar and it is made in a carefully regulated way. One interesting fact about cholesterol is that unlike other fats, our body is not able to use it as a source of energy as we do not have the enzymes needed to break it down.

We are advised to reduce the amount of cholesterol we eat but does the cholesterol in our food have an impact on our cholesterol levels? Around one in five hundred people have a genetic problem that prevents them regulating their cholesterol but everyone else is able to regulate the amount of cholesterol that is circulating. Some of the cholesterol we eat is absorbed in our digestive tract but all experiments that have looked at the consumption of cholesterol rich food have shown that is has only a minor impact on the amount circulating in the blood. Notwithstanding that it was more than sixty years ago Ancel Keys, the man who began the war on fat, is on record as making the statement:

"cholesterol in food has no impact on cholesterol in our blood and we have known that all along "

Despite his war on saturated fat Ancel Keys never withdrew this statement.

When you consider how important cholesterol is to us it is amazing to think that we are being told to reduce our cholesterol levels.

Good and bad cholesterol

Like all fats cholesterol does not dissolve in water, so in order for it to be able to travel around our bodies to the places where it is needed it is packaged up inside proteins that circulate in our blood. These proteins are called lipoproteins, the '*lipo*' bit coming from lipids, the medical name for fats.

Some of us will have heard of 'good' and 'bad' cholesterol. The good guy is HDL cholesterol, High Density Lipoprotein and the bad guy is LDL, Low Density Lipoprotein. However, there is actually no such thing as 'good' or 'bad' cholesterol. Cholesterol is cholesterol. The only difference is the way it is transported around our bodies. As the name suggests, in the HDL cholesterol the cholesterol is carried around in small, dense particles. In the LDL cholesterol the cholesterol is carried around in much bigger particles that are far less dense. Just to add to the confusion about cholesterol there are other lipoproteins that carry other fats like triglycerides and phospholipids around. Very Low Density Lipoproteins, VLDL, and Intermediate Density Lipoproteins, IDL. The VLDL lipoproteins carry mainly triglycerides but they also carry some cholesterol around our bodies.

So why have HDL and LDL cholesterol been labeled as being good and bad? The simplest way of looking at it is that the LDL lipoproteins carry the cholesterol around our body to where it is needed. Because it is transporting it to where it is needed the LDL lipoproteins give up their cholesterol easily. One reason why the LDL lipoproteins are considered to be 'bad' is that they are thought to deposit some of the cholesterol they carry onto the walls of arteries where it can become oxidised and then damage the lining of the arteries. HDL cholesterol carries unused cholesterol back to the liver for recycling. Unlike LDL cholesterol, HDL cholesterol hangs on to the cholesterol it is carrying and in the process of transporting it back to the liver it appears to be able to mop up some of the cholesterol that has been deposited on the walls of arteries.

How much cholesterol does our body need?

The simple answer to this is we do not know. Somehow, in some way and for some reason our body regulates the amount of cholesterol it produces. By taking samples and looking at cholesterol levels across populations scientists can see what is 'normal'. In other words the amount of cholesterol that most people have, but the figure that is normal today could well be very different to the figure that was normal say ten or twenty years ago. When attention was first drawn to the cholesterol and Statin issue America and Australia set target levels for 'bad' LDL cholesterol. In the UK the evidence based medicine body NICE, National Institute for Clinical Excellence did not.

> *"A target for total cholesterol or LDL cholesterol is not recommended for primary prevention of Cardiovascular disease .... NICE does not recommend the use of target levels for people taking Statins for primary prevention of heart disease. This is because it found no clinical trials in primary prevention that have evaluated the relative and absolute benefits of achieving different cholesterol targets in relation to clinical events"*

Despite this statement various medical bodies in the UK took it upon themselves to set levels and these levels were lower than those set by America and Australia.

Cholesterol tests

We are constantly being told that high levels of cholesterol are bad for us and that we need to get our cholesterol checked. If your bad LDL cholesterol is high the medical profession, science and the media are more or less frightening us into lowering it with Statins and plant sterols.

The total amount of cholesterol circulating in your blood depends on the time of day the blood test is taken, whether you have eaten before the blood test was taken, the amount of stress you are under and whether you are low in vitamin D. All of these can affect the results of the test.

When we visit our doctors surgery the test we have measures the total amount of good and bad cholesterol as well as other fats in our blood. It can differentiate between the 'good' HDL cholesterol but all other fats, including triglycerides carried as VLDL, are what is left when we take the HDL from the total. An agreed approximation, called the Friedwald equation, is used to break this figure down into bad LDL cholesterol and triglycerides as VLDL. This is based on the concept that most of the triglycerides carried in the VLDL particles are carried in the ratio of five triglycerides to one cholesterol. So what most people are not aware of is that the standard blood test for cholesterol does not measure bad cholesterol, it estimates it and this is not necessarily a good thing.

The general consensus is that the higher your total and LDL cholesterol levels are the greater your risk of developing cardiovascular disease. But some heart attacks happen when people do not have high levels of LDL cholesterol. As a result some researchers and the National Institute for Clinical Excellence now recommend measuring non HDL cholesterol, the known amount of HDL subtracted from the total amount of cholesterol and other fats in the blood. This gives a better assessment of the risk of heart disease especially if you have high levels of triglycerides.

Statins

Why we were told that diesel engines were less polluting than petrol engines is a mystery, but we know now that it was a fib. Are Statins really as good for us as they are being made out to be or are they like diesel engines another fib?

Statins are possibly the most widely prescribed drug in the world. One in four

Americans over the age of forty five are thought to be taking them. They are also one of the most lucrative drugs in the world. They have earned the pharmaceutical company that developed them around $125 billion since they were first bought to the market in 1997. Now that they are being manufactured by other companies their price has fallen and there are far more around. This inevitably makes it easier for doctors and physicians to prescribe them.

How Statins work

Statins work by inhibiting the production of the enzymes your body needs to make cholesterol. In other words they stop our body making cholesterol. In view of the fact that cholesterol is essential for life and it is something that is so important that our body carefully regulates the amount it produces, this sounds quite drastic.

Do Statins reduce the risk of heart disease? There is some evidence that for people with a history of heart disease taking Statins could reduce the risk of another heart attack. However, this appears not to be because they reduce the levels of cholesterol but because they reduce other risk factors one of which is inflammation. Exercise, losing weight, taking an aspirin each day, eating less inflammatory food or taking an Omega 3 supplement could also reduce inflammation.

So for people with an existing heart condition the evidence is clear. However, one of the largest and most recent studies followed 52,000 men and women in Norway aged between twenty and seventy four for ten years. The study was published in 2011. None of the people in the study had a pre existing heart problem. Surprisingly the results showed that women with low, rather than high, total cholesterol had an increased risk of dying either from a heart attack or other causes. For the men, high cholesterol was associated with heart disease and death from all causes but so also was low cholesterol, low cholesterol being defined as less than 5mmol/L. Interestingly, even though the average cholesterol across the population is between 5mmol/L and 7mmol/L, in the UK 5mmol/L is the maximum recommended level of cholesterol.

When you visit your doctor or medical practitioner your risk of developing cardiovascular disease is usually assessed by them taking into consideration your age, sex, blood pressure, weight and BMI, cholesterol levels, drinking habits, whether or not you smoke and the amount of exercise you get on a regular basis. In the UK a computer programme called QRISK2 is used to make this assessment. Before taking Statins, in the UK the advice from NICE, the National Institute for Clinical Excellence, is to stop smoking, reduce your weight, reduce the amount of alcohol you drink and increase the amount of exercise you take.

An interesting point about the risk assessment is that the 'risk' and the advice whether or not to take Statins has significantly changed over the last twelve years. Up until 2005 Statins were only recommended if you had a 30% or greater risk of having a heart attack in the next ten years. This was later reduced to a 20% risk and then in 2014 NICE came out with a recommendation that the figure should be reduced to a 10% risk of a heart attack in the next ten years because according to NICE:

> *"the price of Stains has fallen, so using Statins to reduce the risk of cardiovascular disease at lower thresholds is now cost effective"*

In other words most men over fifty and most women over sixty should be taking Statins. These updated guidelines created something of an outcry among the scientific and medical professions. In June 2014 a group of doctors and academics published an open letter criticising the independence of NICE and calling on them to withdraw their guidelines on Statins. If you go onto the internet this letter is easy to find.

So is it cost, a cost benefit analysis, high pressure selling by pharmaceutical companies or the well being of the population that is driving the widespread use of Statins? It is an interesting fact that when surveyed, six out of ten general practioners opposed the NICE guidelines and 55% said they would not take Statins themselves.

Side effects of Statins.

One in five of the people taking Statins experience side effects; memory loss, muscle weakness, blurred vision, diarrhoea, disrupted sleep and confusion are just some of them. But one other side effect that is rarely talked about is sexual dysfunction and it is interesting to note that this is also not mentioned in the prescribing information for Statins. Statins reduce the amount of cholesterol we have and cholesterol is needed to make steroid hormones. Testosterone and oestrogen are steroid hormones, so it stands to reason that reducing the amount of cholesterol you have is highly likely to have an adverse effect on them. Men taking Statins are twice as likely to have low levels of testosterone and loss of libido. Many women also report loss of libido but as many women take Statins at the onset of the menopause this side effect is often discounted and attributed to "usual menopausal symptoms".

Statins have been linked to an increased risk of developing type 2 diabetes and in post menopausal women some of the figures that have been published are quite alarming. The higher the dose the greater the risk. A study of men in Finland found that Statins were associated with an almost 50% higher risk of developing type 2 diabetes, even after the data was adjusted for other factors. Statins appear to increase a person's insulin resistance and they also appear to have an adverse impact on the ability of the pancreas to secrete insulin. According to diabetes.co.uk;

> "........... diabetes and Statins have a complex relationship and are the focus of intense patient and health care debate .... it is a complex relationship due to the knowledge that people with diabetes face an increased risk of heart attack and stroke."

As well as inhibiting the production of the enzymes we need to make cholesterol, Statins deplete our body of one of its other enzymes, Coenzyme Q10. This is often referred to as CoQ10. This enzyme is needed by every cell in our body to produce energy in the form of ATP, adenosine triphosphate, and this includes your heart. Adenosine triphosphate is a fundamental part of living and CoQ10 is often referred to as the 'spark plug' that gets things going. The effect Statins have on CoQ10 accounts for the general fatigue and fall in energy levels that some people experience when they take Statins. However, as well as being an enzyme that is needed to produce energy CoQ10 is also a very powerful antioxidant. It is also a mechanism through which vitamin C and vitamin E are reactivated as antioxidants after they have neutralised free radicals. So by reducing the amount of CoQ10 we have available we are reducing our body's armoury of antioxidants and increasing the risk of a state of oxidative stress developing.

So Statins come with side effects, some of which are severe. Does the health benefit to the population outweigh the side effects? Well according to diabetes.co.uk for every thousand people at risk of cardiovascular disease that take Statins for three years, the Statins will prevent seven non fatal heart attacks, four strokes and two deaths. This means that nearly 99% of those taking them will not benefit from Statins but 1% will. With an at risk population of 17.5 million the argument is that thousands of heart attacks, strokes and death could be prevented. However this is not without a very large number of people experiencing major side effects.

Plant sterols

Plant sterols occur naturally in all plants. They are closely related to cholesterol but they are not cholesterol. Cholesterol is only found in animals. In a healthy balanced diet we consume very few plant sterols and as a consequence our body absorbs very few of them. However, polyunsaturated vegetable oils contain much larger amounts of plant sterols than vegetables so when we consume large amounts of food that is fried in vegetable oil we consume and therefore have the opportunity to absorb far more plant sterols. A typical western diet is thought to contain between 400mg and 500mg of plant sterols a day. When plant sterols are added to margarine, low fat spreads, drinks and yogurt we are able to consume yet more of them.

Foods containing plant sterols are being heavily advertised for their cholesterol lowering effects. The current jargon is 'heart healthy' or 'cholesterol busting'. In the UK the current guidelines on plant sterols from NICE is that they do:

"........... not recommend plant sterols in spreads, drinks and yogurts because there is not enough evidence at the moment that these help to prevent cardiovascular disease"

Plant sterols work by competing with cholesterol for absorption in our digestive tract and this is how they are thought to be able to reduce the amount of cholesterol we have in our blood. We absorb the plant sterols in preference to cholesterol. However, when you read between the lines it is clear that they are only thought to work if they are consumed alongside Statins. Plant sterols are known to slightly lower the absorption of fat soluble compounds like vitamin E and the beta carotenes. Precisely what 'slightly lower' means is unclear, but vitamin E and the beta carotenes play an essential role in our antioxidant defences.

While you will see many statements that plant sterols are safe to eat there is actually no evidence that consuming them in amounts that are greater than the amounts that occur naturally in nature is good for us. Like cholesterol they are absorbed into cells and cell membranes, so is their increased consumption like polyunsaturated vegetable oils and trans fats another ticking bomb in terms of our health?

There is no evidence that replacing cholesterol with plant sterols reduces the incidence of cardiovascular disease. There is evidence however, that reducing levels of cholesterol appears to increase and not reduce the incidence of heart disease, stroke and diabetes.

When you look at the small print the sad fact is that a lot of the research into plant sterols and cholesterol is being funded by large food organisations. Because of this we need to be cautious about what we are being told about the results.

Cholesterol, is it friend or foe?

In the war against saturated fat John Yudkin made the observation that saturated fat had been around for thousands of years whereas sugar and refined carbohydrates were a new introduction to our diet. There is absolutely no doubt that the same applies to cholesterol. Cholesterol is essential for human life and it is something that our body regulates. We therefore have to ask ourselves why is cholesterol a problem now? Are levels of cholesterol across populations actually too high or are the target levels that been set as being 'normal' too low? Another more significant question is that if levels of cholesterol are high, why are they high? Is there a reason why our body is making more cholesterol? Well one thing that no one tells you about cholesterol is that it works in tandem with our immune system and this is where the story gets interesting.

Chronic or systemic inflammation increases the risk of just about every serious disease including heart attacks and strokes. Insulin resistance, being overweight and stress all increase inflammation. Scientists have known for many years that atherosclerosis is an inflammatory disease. CRP, C-Reactive Protein, is a measure of inflammation and high levels of CRP have been shown to be a good predictor of the onset of cardiovascular disease. It is well recognised that Statins have an anti inflammatory effect and that they lower CRP.

When our body is in a state of chronic inflammation, oxidative stress, physical stress or trauma, more cells than normal are dying or being damaged. In order to repair them or build new cells cholesterol is needed, it is an essential part of cell walls. Our body is unable to repair or regenerate cells without cholesterol. So the greater the inflammation, the greater the damage to our body, the greater the need for cholesterol. To call LDL cholesterol 'bad' is misleading. It is doing what it is meant to do, take cholesterol to where it is needed. The question that should be asked is why is cholesterol needed in greater amounts than 'normal'. All of our steroid hormones are made from cholesterol and the stress hormone cortisol is one of them. So when we are under emotional stress or suffering from disrupted sleep our body makes more cortisol and in order to do this it needs more cholesterol. Cholesterol levels rise.

When inflammation or something else damages the wall of an artery cholesterol is called to the scene. Without cholesterol the healing process is not possible. Cholesterol provides the fat needed to repair the damaged cell walls or build new cells. When it accumulates on the wall of a blood vessel it can cause narrowing and because it is at the scene of the crime so to speak it is seen as being the culprit, but cholesterol does not cause the damage in the first place. Only time will tell what the real cause of the damage is.

The saturated fat fib has been around for decades but it was recently exposed in a report in the British Journal of Sports Medicine, a division of the British Medical Journal and the BMJ is one of the most highly respected medical journals in the world. In March 2017 the journal published a review of several large studies and it stated that:

> "Despite popular belief among doctors and the public, the conceptual model of dietary saturated fat clogging a pipe is just plain wrong .... Saturated fat does not clog the arteries: coronary heart disease is a chronic inflammatory condition, the risk of which can be effectively reduced from healthy lifestyle interventions ....It is time to shift the public health message in the prevention and treatment of coronary artery disease away from measuring serum lipids and reducing dietary saturated fat. Coronary artery disease is a chronic inflammatory disease and it can be reduced effectively by walking for 20 minutes a day and eating real food. There is no business model or market to help spread this simple yet powerful intervention."

Slowly opinions are beginning to change. If you reduce inflammation cholesterol will take care of itself. What causes inflammation? A diet high in refined carbohydrates, sugar and just about everything made from them and the major disparity between Omega 3 and Omega 6 polyunsaturated vegetable oils that occurs in the typical western diet. The more refined carbohydrates and sugar consumed the greater the inflammation and the higher the cholesterol. The more Omega 6 fats in the form of polyunsaturated vegetable oils and trans fats consumed the greater the inflammation and the higher the cholesterol. High levels of cholesterol are in reality a wakeup call that is telling us that all is not well. While for some an under active thyroid can be the cause, for most people the real problem is more likely to be chronic inflammation and this is something that we can all do something about.

The whole issue of saturated fats, Cholesterol, Statins and plant sterols is shrouded in myths and received wisdom and none of this is supported by facts. Somehow and in some way science and medicine have made cholesterol into a villain, yet there is no evidence to support this view. We need to look at the big picture and take a holistic view of what cholesterol is and why we need it. Finding the truth will not be easy.

Conclusion

Here we have the five big fibs about food and together they have had a devastating impact on the food we eat, our weight and our health. Cholesterol, Statins and plant sterols may in the course of time prove to be another fib and it could possibly be the biggest fib of them all. While it may not make us fat it could be the most damaging all in terms of our health.

So if you are what you eat what should we be eating? Which foods are good to eat, which foods are not so good and which foods are just plain bad? May be if we take a step back and take a look at history we will be able to find some clues.

Chapter Four

What Is A Healthy Diet?

Do our ancestors tell us anything

Modern humans evolved about two and a half million years ago. The agricultural revolution began around 10,000 years ago. Prior to the agricultural revolution all humans lived as hunter gatherers. They obtained their food by foraging, hunting and fishing. With the advent of the agricultural revolution grains like wheat, rice and corn were domesticated and food became more plentiful and more readily available. Cattle and sheep were domesticated and people began drinking milk. More babies were born and reared successfully and populations exploded. Ironically there is clear archaeological evidence that when this happened, rather than becoming bigger and healthier, people became shorter and the general state of their health declined. The people who continued to live as hunter gatherers were either assimilated into the agricultural communities or pushed off of the productive land into remote areas.

What do we know about what our early ancestors ate before the Agricultural revolution? Well over the years paleo anthropologists have learned a surprising amount. Received wisdom tells us that it was hunting and the consumption of large amounts of meat that made us human. However, the archaeological evidence tells us otherwise. Meat is an energy rich food and there is no doubt that meat, and to a lesser extent fish, played a key role in our early evolution. But contrary to what we have been led to believe our early ancestors probably obtained at most only about 30% of their calories from meat. The rest came from a wide diversity of plants, roots, tubers, nuts, seeds, fruit, honey and in coastal areas significant amounts of shell fish that were foraged. Rather than just eating meat, what appears to have made us human was our ability to adapt to our environment and find a meal more or less anywhere.

Over recent years Paleo and Primal diets have become increasingly popular. As these diets are based on the premise that as a species we stopped evolving in the Paleolithic period and only began eating grains during the Agricultural revolution, are they a good blueprint for a modern diet? Well, the notion that we stopped evolving in the Paleolithic period is actually not true. Paleo biologists have found plenty of evidence to the contrary. It is also clear that we have been eating grains and tubers for well over 100,000 years.

They were eaten in small amounts and they were eaten whole and totally unrefined, but they were clearly part of our early diet.

In evolutionary terms the 10,000 years since the agricultural revolution is a very short time, but we know that we did evolve in order to be able to digest the food that farming made available to us. We also adapted in various other ways to a non hunter gatherer diet. Because the DNA inside each of our cells controls which enzymes our bodies make and hence the food we are able to digest, studies of ancient DNA have cast some light on what our ancestors were able to eat. Some populations evolved with changes to enzymes that made them better able to deal with starchy foods, some developed the enzymes needed to process the alcohol found in fermented foods and some developed the enzymes needed to digest milk. The ability to digest milk and dairy products is a striking example of how our DNA has changed. All humans are born with the ability to digest their mothers milk, but before the agricultural revolution, when children were weaned they lost this ability because there was no milk to drink, they did not need it any more. So as adults they were lactose intolerant. Enter the agricultural revolution and the domestication of cattle and sheep, having the ability to digest milk gave us a new protein rich food and a tremendous advantage. As a result lactose tolerance evolved in the groups of people that reared cattle but not in people like the Chinese and south east Asians who did not rear them.

Are there any 'living fossils' that we can study?

The answer is yes, but they are disappearing fast. By the year 2050 there will be two billion more people on this planet that need to be fed. This gives the question of what these people should be eating a level of urgency, simply because the food we choose to eat over the forthcoming years will have a profound impact on the health and welfare of our planet. If these people eat the current 'Western Diet' of meat and refined grains it will take a far greater toll on the world's environment and resources than a diet that revolves around vegetables, nuts, fruits, unrefined grains and possibly even insects.

Because of the pressure on the earth's food resources scientists are particularly interested in learning about the diets of the few indigenous hunter gatherer peoples that remain isolated from the developed world. Their diet could not only cast some light on what the rest of us should be eating but also show us how their health changes as they move away from their traditional diet and lifestyle and adopt the eating habits of the developed countries. So far the studies that have been undertaken reveal that irrespective of what their diet is, when these people are in their natural environment they are not overweight, they do not develop high blood pressure and they do not suffer from diabetes, atherosclerosis or cardiovascular disease. They only get into trouble when they abandon their traditional diets and active lifestyles and adopt the eating habits of the west.

Like our early ancestors most of the hunter gatherers that remain today obtain around 70% of their calories from plants, nuts, seeds and tubers. Year round observations confirm that even with traps, nets, spears, bows and arrows hunter gatherers often have only limited success in obtaining meat. Half the time they come home empty handed and when they do manage to bring back meat there is often only just enough to go round.

It is clear that there is a tremendous variation in what food we as humans can thrive on. Some diets are lacto vegetarian, some are based only on plants, some are based on meat and some are based on fish and seafood. It makes sense that our evolutionary history and genetic inheritance goes some way to explaining how we deal with the food we eat and why some people thrive and others fail to flourish when eating the same food. Because of this most scientists agree that there is no one ideal human diet. Our ability to adapt and combine many different foods to create a healthy diet is key to our success as a species. Sadly the typical Western diet does not appear to be one of the healthy ones.

The golden cohort

It is only in relatively recent history that excess weight began to affect all the social classes. In the UK a public health report published in 1923 made the observation that excess weight was only an issue for the middle and upper classes. Working class people generally were not overweight, probably because they could only afford a basic near subsistence diet. Then along came World War II and in 1940 in the UK the introduction of rationing. Rationing continued for 14 years and it changed the eating habits of a generation. Ironically this lead to a healthier population. Irrespective of how much money you had to spend, with the exception of food obtained on the black market, everyone had to have the same amount of food.

In 2011 a study in the UK by the Office of National Statistics showed that there was a 'golden cohort' of people, born between the late 1920's and late 1930's, who were enjoying longer and healthier lives than their predecessors and those born after them. The implication was that their health and longevity was somehow linked to them having grown up with rationing in their formative years

Is there anything we can learn from this in terms of what a healthy diet should be? Most of us think of war time rationing as a 'near starvation diet' but the actual daily calorie value was around 3,000 calories, up to 1,000 calories more than we are recommended today. Two things that were not rationed were vegetables and fruit. Today only 30% of us eat the recommended 'five a day' and this is far less than our war time counterparts would have consumed. This war time diet of vegetables and seasonal fruit combined with oatmeal, usually in the form of porridge, and whole grain bread in the form of the 'national loaf' delivered nearly double the amount of fibre we consume today. Weekly sugar rations were less than half of what most of us consume today and because meat was rationed by price cheaper cuts and far more offal were consumed. Paradoxically these cheaper cuts of meat contained far more saturated fat than the leaner more expensive cuts.

Did the population of war time Britain eat vegetable oils? No because they were not widely available and olive oil was only used for medicinal purposes. Fat from meat was saved, clarified and used for cooking and because it was in short supply it was used sparingly. Did they eat margarine? Very little. Like meat margarine was rationed by price. Of the two types of margarine available the 'value' brand was not very palatable and the up market quality version was actually quite expensive. Did they eat processed food? In the 1940's the humble British sausage, the 'banger', and tins of Spam imported from America was the closest most people got to food that was in any way processed.

The Grain Debate

Since the agricultural revolution grains and cereals have provided more and more of our food. Over recent years consumption has soared. Today edible grains make up the majority of the world's cultivated crops and after sugar they provide the biggest percentage of the calories consumed worldwide.

There is no doubt that as well as having the potential to cause allergies and food sensitivities, wheat and most other cereal grains are acidic inflammatory foods. The more hybridised and processed the grain is the greater its inflammatory potential. Whole grains are the least inflammatory of the grains but in some people they can still trigger an adverse immune reaction, particularly in people suffering from coeliac disease.

Grains and cereals are now in the middle of a sort of public relations nightmare with people claiming major health benefits by adopting grain free diets. Some people actually go as far as to say that grains and cereals are toxic. Are grains good for us or are they bad? Well, all grains and cereals contain things that could potentially be bad for us. As well as the protein gluten, most grains and cereals also contain compounds called anti-nutrients, substances that can interfere with our ability to absorb minerals and trace elements like calcium, iron and manganese. Some advocates of a grain free diet believe that these anti nutrients act as toxins in our bodies. However, almost all food derived from plants contain anti nutrients in one form or another as they are the plants' natural defence against pests, diseases and environmental threats. Tubers like potatoes are no exception. Many tubers are relatively toxic if eaten raw and a green potato, even when cooked, is actually quite poisonous.

The three anti nutrients that are often singled out are phytates in the form of phytic acid, lectins and trypsin inhibitors as they are thought to impair or damage the lining of the intestine and lead to digestive problems and food sensitivities. However, all three of these are present in varying amounts in all plant based foods. Most of them are deactivated and become harmless when they are cooked, but some can still be active when we eat them. Interestingly, the lectin usually found in grains and cereals is not completely deactivated by cooking. Notwithstanding this, foods like apples, bananas and carrots all contain lectins and we eat most of these raw. As with so many things lectins and the other anti nutrients probably become an issue when they are consumed too often and in large amounts.

In the grain debate gluten is a key issue as it is known to be an allergen that can cause severe inflammation in the small minority of people who are unable to digest it. About 1% of the population of the developed world suffer from coeliac disease, an allergic auto immune condition that is associated with the consumption of grains like wheat and barley that contain gluten. True coeliac disease and gluten allergy at one end of the spectrum only affects a small minority of people but at the other end of the spectrum there are people who are sensitive to but not actually allergic to gluten. Notwithstanding this the sensitivity can create an inflammatory response. Unlike coeliac disease gluten sensitivity does not have any biomarkers so it can only be diagnosed by first ruling out other diseases and then trying a gluten free diet. Some researchers on gluten sensitivity estimate that around 6% of people of European decent have some degree of gluten sensitivity. It is worth bearing in mind that not all grains contain gluten; amaranth, buckwheat, corn, millet, most oats, quinoa and rice are all gluten free so should they be excluded from the grain debate?

The consumption of grains and cereals is fast becoming a big issue. Part of the controversy about going gluten free and gluten sensitivity is that we are being sold a great deal of misinformation. Several best selling books have been highly influential in steering healthy people away from the 'dangers' of wheat and gluten by making generalisations and exaggerated claims. Some go as far as to say that gluten and carbohydrates are destroying our brains!

Some prominent people have treated genuine physiological conditions themselves by excluding gluten from their diet and the media coverage has meant that their stories have snowballed. Now more and more people are taking the view that '*if it works for them it must be worth giving it a go*'. Enter the placebo effect and for many it becomes difficult to disentangle the benefits they may experience by adopting a gluten free diet from their expectation that the change in their diet will make them feel better.

The bottom line is that with the typical western diet we push our bodies too far. If you suspect that you are sensitive to a specific food or group of foods try eliminating it for at least two weeks. Listen to your body and see if symptoms like lethargy, headaches, 'foggy mind', depression, flatulence or bloating subside. Tedious and time consuming it may be but it is worth it in the long term. One last thing about food sensitivities is that as we get older foods that never bothered us before, like dairy and wheat, may trigger chronic low grade indigestion or other seemingly minor symptoms that can put our immune system onto high alert.

If you do decide to try an exclusion diet be mindful that they are not risk free. Many people with eating disorders begin with an exclusion diet that spirals out of control. The end result is anxiety and stress, both of which are entirely counter productive to your overall state of health.

The grain debate is having a major impact on public opinion which, according to market research company Mintel, is split between 41% of people in the United States who think that gluten free diets are of benefit and 44% who think they are a fad. A recent survey found that 29% of adult Americans, 70 million people, were trying to cut back on their consumption of gluten. In the UK the polster YouGov reported that 60% of adults have at some time purchased a gluten free product and that 10% of households, over 2½ million homes, include someone who believes that gluten is bad for them.

Enter the food manufacturing industry which has quickly cottoned on to 'gluten free' as being the latest marketing ploy, with projected revenue in the United States estimated to increase from $8.8bn in 2014 to $14.2bn in 2017. In the UK new product launches of 'healthy' gluten free snack bars has increased from 25% in 2013 to 40% in 2014.

Why have our views on the consumption of grains changed so rapidly? Some people have suggested that the increased interest in a gluten free diet has little to do with public awareness of coeliac disease and gluten sensitivity but a lot to do with the popularity of diets that are aimed at moving us back to the type of hunter gatherer food our early ancestors are thought to have consumed. Others see it as connecting these myths about man's early diet with an increasing "anti" attitude to the food manufacturing industry. One thing is certain however, with the food manufacturing industry now focused on a new rapidly growing sector, with increased advertising and promotional activity "gluten free" and the grain debate is destined to become an even bigger hot topic and possibly yet another food fib.

Are we simply eating too many grains?

The ability to grow and process grains and cereals more easily allowed people to eat more of them, but the change in our consumption of grains and cereals has not happened over the thousands of years since the agricultural revolution. Up until fairly recent history only the rich could afford to eat flour that was in any way refined and even then it was far less refined than our current 'white' flour. As you went down through the social scale less wheat and more rye and oatmeal were consumed and the coarser and less refined this 'flour' became. By the time you got to the really poor, they could not afford flour at all. They ate a sort of meal made from ground up beans and pulses, the equivalent of current day gram or chickpea flour.

While we may have the enzymes needed to digest them, from an evolutionary perspective the 10,000 years since the Agricultural Revolution is no where near long enough for our digestive systems to have evolved enough to be able to cope with the enormous amounts of highly refined grains and cereals that we have in our diet today. The bottom line is that we are simply eating too many grains and cereals and the ones we are eating are in the wrong form; refined grains for breakfast in our cereal, refined grains for lunch in some form of bread, may be a muffin at some time of the day as a snack and probably more refined grains in the evening as pasta or pizza.

The jury is still out on the grain debate. It depends to a certain extent on which side of the fence you are sitting. Consuming grains and cereals may be right for some people and wrong for others. When you do eat them focus on quality, eat smaller amounts and only eat 'whole' complex grains. Eat more vegetables and non grain sources of carbohydrates like pulses whenever you can. Eating a balanced diet and cutting back on something that everyone agrees is being consumed in amounts that are far too large can only be a good thing.

The Meat Debate

Many people eating a typical western diet consume meat at every meal of the day. Studies of our early ancestors and the hunter gatherers that are left in their natural environment show that "man the carnivore" is actually something of a myth. The hunter gatherers that have been observed obtain only about 30% of their calories from meat. They do not eat meat every day, they eat it only when it is available and there is no reason to assume that our early ancestors were any different.

Meat is clearly an important part of our diet, human beings are omnivores, but how much meat should we be eating? We all know that meat provides us with a valuable source of protein, fat and vitamins and it also provides us with iron. Iron and the type of fats in meat could provide us with a clue about how much meat is too much.

Iron is an essential nutrient and for years a lack of it caused one of the most common nutritional deficiencies, anaemia. However, in the Western world more attention is being paid these days to the opposite problem, iron overload. Iron is essential for life. It is used to transport oxygen around our body. It is used in the conversion of sugar into adenosine triphosphate, the store of energy inside each of our cells, and it is needed to make catalase, one of the important antioxidants our body makes. However, despite its importance it would appear that high levels of iron can sometimes cause problems and interestingly 'iron overload' has been linked to an increased risk of diabetes, coronary heart disease and some cancers.

Our body handles iron very carefully, to the extent that it even recycles it from red blood cells that have died. Recycling is essential as, like the hunter gatherers that remain, the human diet historically contained only just enough iron to replace the small amount that is lost each day. A hormone called hepcidin enables our body to regulate the 'uptake' of iron; the less iron you have the more iron your body absorbs, likewise the more iron you have the less it absorbs. Because iron is so important our body guards its store of iron very carefully, so carefully in fact that it has no way of excreting it. Each day we only need a trace amount of iron to replace the tiny amount that we lose. Even for an adult man this is as little as 1mg to 2mg a day. Because our body is unable to completely shut down the absorption process the more iron we consume and absorb from our food the higher the level of stored iron becomes. Short of a blood donation, our body is unable to get rid of it.

In a 10 year study of 32,000 women, those who consumed the most iron, and as a consequence had the highest levels of stored iron, were nearly three times more likely to have insulin resistance and type 2 diabetes than those with the lowest levels of iron. In another study of 38,000 men, those who consumed the most iron had a 63% greater risk of developing type 2 diabetes. Now this begs the question of whether is it the actual iron or other things in the food containing the iron that was causing the diabetes. It could also be that other foods consumed with the iron rich food, a steak with chips or fries for instance, were contributing to the problem. However, other studies have since shown that when people with high levels of stored iron donate blood on a regular basis, their insulin sensitivity and risk of diabetes diminishes. Why? Put simply the current thinking is that iron overload damages the pancreas and affects its ability to produce insulin, so the end result for some is insulin resistance and type 2 diabetes.

Where Does The Iron In Our Diet Come From?

Meat, fish, poultry, eggs and vegetables all contain iron. However, there are two different types of iron. HEME iron is a type of iron that is derived from red blood cells and it is only found in meat, fish and poultry. Non HEME iron is found in vegetables and fruit as well as animal products. The HEME iron found in meat is much more easy to absorb than non HEME iron. Whereas between 15% and 30% of HEME iron is absorbed, only about 5% of non HEME iron finds its way into our blood. Interestingly, the uptake of the iron from vegetables is much better regulated by the body than the uptake of the iron from meat, so the accumulation of iron and iron 'over load' is more likely if your diet is high in the HEME iron found in animal products.

Various factors can influence the way in which iron is absorbed and not least of these is gender. Pre menopausal women absorb iron much more efficiently than men; from a similar meal they will absorb around three times as much as a man and when a woman is pregnant this figure can increase to around nine times. Vitamin C, some of the proteins found in meat, and acids naturally present in many fruits and vegetables can all increase the absorption of the non HEME iron found in vegetables, sometimes by as much as 85%. Interestingly alcohol and sugar consumption enhance the absorption of both types of iron. While Vitamin C has a neutral effect on how the iron from animal products is absorbed, the anti nutrients that are in some vegetables can interfere with and slow down the absorption of the iron. So it would appear that the more vegetables and fibre you eat the less iron from animal products your body is able to take on board. Where else does the iron in our diet come from? Probably as a legacy from the past, when dietary iron was in short supply, most manufactured food is now enriched with iron; flour, breakfast cereals, breads, pasta, even infant formula and baby foods are all fortified with iron and many of us also take daily vitamin supplements without realising that they also often contain iron.

Are we eating too much meat?

Not so long ago, before meat farming became the semi industrialised process it is today, the price of meat and poultry was high. Only the wealthy could afford to eat it every day. For most people meat was something of a luxury that was only consumed once or twice a week and even then, it was only consumed in modest amounts. However, with the advent of intensive farming methods the price of meat dropped and as a consequence consumption has soared. In 1961 the world's total meat supply was estimated to be 71 million tons. By 2007, it had risen to 284 million tons. When you allow for world population growth and real changes in global GDP, this represents a 70% increase. Per capita consumption has more than doubled over that period. In developing countries it has risen twice as fast, doubling in the last 20 years.

Americans are now consuming close to 276 pounds of meat, poultry and fish per person per year and getting on for half of this is red meat. Australians are consuming almost as much but in Luxembourg the figure is even higher; 300lbs or just over 140kg per person per year. Not surprisingly India has the lowest consumption of meat at 7 pounds, just over 3 kg a person. The consumption of 276 pounds of meat a year works out at just under 12 ounces or 350 grams of meat, poultry or fish a day. Red meat contains around 3.7mg iron per 100 grams, fish and poultry around 1.3mg. So if you consume 350 grams of animal protein a day that's just under 13mg from red meat and 4½mg from poultry and fish. As getting on for half of our animal protein consumption is from red meat, that averages out at around 8¾mg of iron a day.

How much iron do we need on a daily basis?

Well, we know that a healthy man only actually needs between 1mg and 2mg of iron a day, so to allow for the fact that not all of the iron we consume is absorbed the recommended daily guideline is 8mg a day for men and post menopausal women and 18mg a day for pre menopausal women. When you look at these figures 8¾mg a day from animal protein doesn't look too bad. However, other foods like bread, breakfast cereals, flour and pasta are all fortified with iron. Because so many nutrients are taken out in the milling and refining process, in most countries white bread is fortified with enough iron to bring it to within 80% of the amount of iron that is naturally found in whole grain bread, 3.6mg per 100 grams. The fibre and phytic acid in whole grain bread reduces the absorption of iron, so this amount of iron isn't too much of a problem, but in white bread there is very little fibre and the phytic acid is removed in the milling process. An average slice of white bread weighs around 70 grams and that gives you 2½mg of iron.

How much bread does the average person consume each day? A lot more than one slice. Breakfast cereal contains anything upwards of 10mg of iron per 100 grams. Even with the recommended serving of just 30 grams this means that 3.3mg of iron are added to the daily iron load and many of us actually eat portions of breakfast cereal that are nearer to 50 or 70 grams. If you include bread, pasta, the occasional muffin and other fortified foods it is easy to see how the recommended daily allowance for iron of 8mg a day is easily exceeded. Just one average portion of animal protein, 2 slices of white bread and 30 grams of breakfast cereal will deliver just over 19mg, more than twice the recommended daily amount. How much of this iron is actually absorbed is another matter as it depends on what other food you are eating, but it is clear that with such an abundant supply of iron slowly, over a number of years, it is easy for iron to accumulate to a level that can potentially cause health problems. So with the widespread consumption of large quantities of animal proteins, iron enriched processed foods and a diet that is low in vegetables, fruit and fibre, many people in the Western world now have levels of stored iron that are higher than they should be and this iron increases the risk of developing insulin resistance and type 2 diabetes.

When iron behaves badly

But the story does not end here. Iron is essential for human life. As well as our red blood cells, amongst other things it is also needed to make catalase, one of the antioxidants our body makes. However, because iron is so important to us it has a selective advantage when it competes with trace elements and minerals like zinc, copper and manganese for absorption. As a consequence it is easy for us to become saturated with iron at the expense of other trace elements and we end up not having enough of them. As iron is needed to make catalase some of the trace elements are needed to make some of the other antioxidants our body makes and when this happens too much iron can cause these antioxidants to be in short supply. One of these antioxidants is a compound called Superoxide Dismutase which is used to mop up free radicals of superoxide. Superoxide free radicals are being constantly produced as part of our normal every day life. Our body needs zinc and copper to make Superoxide Dismutase and if these are in short supply some of the superoxide free radicals can go unchecked.

The HEME and non HEME iron we consume in our food is in the form of particles called 'ions'. Like free radicals these are highly active and unstable so they need to attach themselves to other compounds in order to make themselves inactive. Vitamin C and a compound in our body called uric acid are able to do this and the anthocyanins and polyphenols that are present in some of the fruit and vegetables we eat are also able to make these ions inactive. However, if there is not enough of these compounds around some of the iron ions remain unstable and they can then react with free radicals to produce some of the most dangerous free radicals our body is exposed to.

Our body produces superoxide and another free radical called hydrogen peroxide in several ways and under normal balanced conditions these two free radicals rarely interact. However, in the presence of some metal ions, particularly iron ions, they can work together in a chain reaction that produces compounds called hydroxyl free radicals. These have a very short life, they work at a localised level and they are highly reactive. This makes them very dangerous compounds that are known to damage DNA and cell membranes. They can also react with any hydrogen peroxide that is left in another chain reaction that produces yet more free radicals, this time in the form of compounds called peroxyl radicals. These hydroxyl and peroxyl free radicals can not be eliminated by any of our body's antioxidants on their own. They need a hefty team of dietary antioxidants to work alongside them in order to make these free radicals safe.

So iron overload can lead to the generation of some very dangerous free radicals that can damage cells and DNA and ultimately either induce a state of oxidative stress or make oxidative stress that already exists worse.

The quality of the meat we eat

In terms of quality the meat and poultry we are eating today has come a long way from the meat and poultry that was eaten 100 years ago. With the intensive farming methods now being used it is hardly surprising that quality has fallen dramatically. Most commercially produced meat and poultry is from animals reared in sheds or pens and even fish is now farmed in large quantities. Instead of feeding on grass, cattle are now kept in pens and fed on corn, soya and grain, pigs no longer root around fields eating their natural omnivorous diet and chickens no longer scratch around eating whatever they can find. As a consequence the nutritional content of the meat, fish and eggs from industrially reared animals is very different to the meat, fish and eggs from animals reared in their natural environment.

Grazing animals convert grass that we cannot eat into meat, a food that we can eat and they convert grass into meat very efficiently. Intensively reared animals that are fed on soya, corn and grain are fed on food that we can eat and they convert it into meat very inefficiently. So to speed up the process they are given growth hormones and because they are kept in very confined spaces where they become sick they are given antibiotics. In the meantime there are millions of people around the world who do not have enough to eat and they could be eating the corn, soya and grain being fed to the animals. Almost universally there are subsidies for the corn, soya and grain that is being fed to intensively reared animals so the price of the meat they produce is much lower than the meat from grass fed animals where there are no subsidies. So meat from intensively reared animals is cheap and readily available. We can more or less eat as much of it as we like.

The idiom "*You are what you eat*" certainly holds true here. Organic free range eggs have a much healthier Omega 3 to Omega 6 ratio than eggs from battery hens, even when the battery hens have been fed on fish meal so that they lay 'Omega 3 enriched' eggs. While the difference in the overall fat content of meat from intensively reared and grass fed cattle is usually only about 5%, the difference in the type of fat in these animals is very significant. Depending on breed, grass fed beef has between two and five times the amount of Omega 3 than grain fed beef and considerably more antioxidants, vitamins and minerals. Why is this important? It is all about the large amounts of Omega 6 that industrially reared animals contain. As with polyunsaturated vegetable fats the large amount of Omega 6 in the meat has the effect of disrupting the balance between the

Omega 3 and Omega 6 fats and because the Omega 6 fats are pro inflammatory this effectively makes the grain fed meat inflammatory. Add to this the potentially adverse impact of the hormones and antibiotics these animals are fed on and you do not have a very healthy product.

How Much Meat Should We Eat

Just about everyone working in the field of nutrition agree that in general, those of us who are eating a typical western, diet are eating far too much meat. We need to eat protein but we do not need a large portion of meat to provide it, and we certainly do not need to make it a part of every meal. Notwithstanding our own health, the health of our planet is suffering as it takes a large amount of resource to provide a kilogramme of meat for human consumption.

Irrespective of whether animals are grass fed or intensively reared there is nowhere near enough land available to provide the amount of meat our appetites are demanding. Cattle grazing is taking a tremendous toll on the environment. In the western states of America it is destroying vegetation, eroding topsoil, displacing wildlife and polluting water. In the Amazon rain forest around 80% of the deforestation is either due to grazing cattle or the need to grow crops to feed intensively reared cattle. Loss of forest is having an enormous impact on greenhouse gases. Growing corn, soya and grain for cattle involves the use of fertilisers and pesticides and unless grass fed cattle are certified as being 'organically reared' fertilisers and pesticides will have been used on their grazing land. All grazing animals produce methane and nitrous oxide gases. In terms of greenhouse gases methane is twenty times more damaging than carbon dioxide. Grass fed cattle are between four and five years old when they reach our table whereas intensively reared cattle are ready in just over a year.

When you consider the time it takes to rear an animal and the amount of greenhouse gas this produces, the amount of grazing land it needs and the amount of land needed to grow the corn, soya and grain the animal is fed on, which is the more environmentally friendly way of rearing animals?

One other thing that needs to be considered in the meat debate is the type of meat we eat. For most of us meat means muscle meat but not so long ago, because meat was in relative terms expensive, all of the animal was consumed. Cheap fatty cuts and 'Awful

Offal' like liver, kidney, tripe, sweetbreads, heart, tongue and charcuterie are packed full of healthy fat and vitamins but today very few of us eat them. They have become part of the 60% of an animal that is 'abattoir waste' and this waste has to be disposed of. Yet another environmental problem for planet earth.

If we are not eating meat where does our protein come from? Eggs have the highest bio availability and surprisingly fish has a higher bio availability than beef. Poultry follows closely behind beef. In the UK the best advice from the National Health Service is to limit the amount of red meat you eat to 70 grams a day. If you are eating 90 grams or more they strongly advise cutting down because

> "............. best evidence shows that there is probably a link between eating meat and bowel cancer".

The words 'best evidence' and 'probably' are interesting and it is all to do with dioxins. Dioxins are a group of chemically related compounds that are persistent environmental pollutants, often referred to as POP's, Persistent Organic Pollutants. They are found throughout the world and they accumulate in the food chain, mainly in the fatty tissue of animals. Around 90% of the dioxins we are exposed to come from our food, meat, dairy, fish and shellfish being the main culprits.

Dioxins are chemically very stable and once they enter our body they are absorbed into our fat tissue where they hang around for a long time. It takes around ten years for our body to get rid of them. Dioxins are known to be highly toxic and they have been linked to a wide range of health problems. Cancer and damage to our immune system are just two of them. Due to their highly toxic nature over the last twenty years steps have been taken to clean up industrial sources of dioxins and reduce our exposure to them, but they are and always will be around us.

Our exposure to dioxins is a big issue and it is a highly complex issue as our exposure comes from natural as well as industrial sources. In urban areas back yard fires are now thought to be a major source of dioxin pollution. In line with this in autumn 2016 the World Health Organisation updated their fact sheet on the effect dioxins have on our health. How much you should worry about dioxins is a personal matter. It is a fact that our exposure to them has reduced over the last twenty years but it is also a fact that they accumulate in our bodies and have the ability to cause serious damage. Different types of food exposes us to different amounts of dioxins and as meat, and in particular fatty meat, is one of the worst culprits it makes sense to cut down on the amount of meat you eat. In other words do not have meat with every meal, eat it in smaller amounts and eat it as part of a balanced diet.

The Way We Cook Our Food

Can cooking methods damage our health? One of the most intriguing aspects of our modern western diet is the high heat at which so much of our food is cooked. We fry food in oil, we grill it, we BBQ it and we roast and bake it in hot ovens. The effect that these cooking methods have on our food is immense. None of the food we eat, irrespective of whether it is of animal or plant origin, is able to withstand cooking at such high temperatures and as a consequence its nutritional content and chemical structure both suffer.

Why do we cook food?

While some food can be eaten in its raw natural state sometimes cooking is needed. It is interesting that as a species it is very difficult for us to thrive on raw food alone. Some scientists believe that the two biggest revolutions in human development came when we learned how to ferment food and how to cook food. Both fermenting and cooking have the effect of 'predigesting' food and enabling us to extract more nutrients and energy from it. They also have the effect of making food safe by killing off dangerous bacteria, tenderising food that would otherwise be tough and unpleasant to eat and increasing the time the food can be kept for. Cooking sometimes also has the benefit of improving the taste and flavour of food and making it look more appetising.

Does cooking produce damaging substances?

Nutritional research is only just starting to catch up with the consequences of our high temperature cooking methods and our addiction to 'browned', 'caramelised' and 'crisp' foods. We know that when oils are heated they oxidise and produce free radicals. The higher the temperature the greater the number of free radicals. But this isn't the only thing that happens. Cooking food at high temperatures, even in the absence of oil, can generate compounds that can cause serious damage to our cells and the DNA within the cells. Aldehydes, Heterocyclic amines (HCA's), polycyclic aromatic hydrocarbons (PAH's),

Acrylamide and Advanced Glycation End Products (AGE's) are just some of these compounds and their consumption has been linked to an enormous number of diseases. Advanced Glycation End products in particular are thought to be a major factor in some age related degenerative diseases and they are known to be linked to insulin resistance, type 2 diabetes and oxidative stress.

What are AGE's and where do they come from?

Advanced Glycation End products come from two sources, our bodies and our food. Our bodies produce them as part of normal metabolism. Carbohydrates, irrespective of whether they are simple or complex, are metabolised into glucose and used by our body as a source of energy. However, a small amount of this glucose is glycated to form AGE's. As we get older AGE's are produced in greater numbers and they are also produced in greater numbers if we have higher than normal amounts of glucose in our blood. Scientists studying diabetes have known about the existence of AGE's for years. They have also known that fructose is glycated ten times faster than glucose. With the dramatic increase in the consumption of sugar and High Fructose Corn Syrup the number of people with high levels of AGE's has increased dramatically over recent years.

Dietary AGE's form as food browns during cooking, primarily when foods high in protein or fat are subjected to high temperatures. When you fry a piece of steak or cook it under the grill you are creating a chemical reaction called a Maillard reaction. This occurs when some of the sugars, fats and proteins in the food react together when they are exposed to high temperatures. The end result are glycotoxins or Advanced Glycation End products. While cooking in dry heat produces the most AGE's, pasteurisation, smoking and microwaving food all produce them. Because the beans from which they are made are roasted even coffee and chocolate contain them. The higher the roasting temperature and the longer the roasting time the more AGE's a food contains. Any food that contains sugars, fats and proteins is fair game. One of the worrying things about AGE's is that for most of us the browning effect they come from enhances the flavour of food. As a consequence they increase our appetite and this encourages us to eat more. It is not surprising that the food manufacturing industry has taken this interesting characteristic on board and now adds sugar in various forms to certain foods in order to enhance their colour and flavour and entice us to eat more; bread, biscuits, baked goods, ready meals and colas all contain them.

Why should we worry about AGE's?

Once inside our body AGE's can damage cells, tissues and organs and this damage causes increased levels of inflammation. They can also accelerate the on set of degenerative diseases. It is estimated that the standard American diet now contains between 10,000 and 16,000 kU of AGEs each day. This is three times higher than the safety limit advised by professional organisations. Most scientists agree that about ten per cent of the AGE's in our food are absorbed and of this 10%, it takes about three days for the body to excrete around a third of them. The remaining two thirds are not excreted. This means that as they slowly accumulate, there are plenty left hanging around in the body to cause trouble.

What can we do about them?

Different foods produce different amounts of AGE's and different cooking methods also create different amounts. For example, if you fry, grill or roast a 90 gram chicken breast it will generate between 4,000 to 9,000 units of AGE's. If you steam, boil or braise it it will produce about 1,000. As a general rule, because they contain less protein, vegetables produce fewer AGE's than animal based products. The more raw foods we eat the lower the number of AGE's. Interestingly, lemon juice and vinegar used as marinades reduces the amount of AGE's that are generated when the food is cooked. So by changing cooking methods, marinading your meat and fish in lemon juice or vinegar and eating less animal protein we can reduce the amount of AGE's we are exposing our bodies to.

To fry or not to fry?

Frying food in polyunsaturated vegetable oils produces compounds called aldehydes. These are extremely damaging substances and consuming or inhaling them even in small amounts has been linked to cancer, cardiovascular disease and degenerative diseases. So the simple answer to this question is not to fry your food, particularly as all fried food is highly inflammatory. Changing the habits of a life time is no easy matter so in reality for most people the best advice is to limit your consumption of fried food to 'once in a while'.

If we accept the fact that we are going to fry food which oils and fats should we be using?

When any oil or fat is heated the oil oxidises and free radicals are produced, often in large numbers. Some of these are very aggressive free radicals that can set off chain reactions that have the potential to cause severe damage to cells. The need to neutralise these free radicals puts an increased load on our body's antioxidant defences.

The more polyunsaturated the fat or oil is the more it oxidises. The more saturated the fat is the less it oxidises. For years we have been told that frying with vegetable oils is healthier than frying with saturated fats like butter or lard, but is it? Oils like sunflower and corn oil that are rich in polyunsaturates generate the highest levels of aldehydes when they are used for frying. In contrast olive oil, butter, lard, coconut oil and goose fat produce far less aldehydes. The reason for this is that these oils are richer in saturated and monounsaturated fatty acids than the polyunsaturated oils. The monounsaturated and saturated fats are much more stable when they are heated. In fact saturated fats generate hardly any aldehydes when they are heated.

Corn oil and sunflower oil are loaded with polyunsaturated fats; corn oils contains 54% and sunflower oil 65%. While it contains 63% monounsaturated fats rape seed oil also contains 28% polyunsaturated fats and these are not in a particularly good Omega 3 to Omega 6 ratio. So the general recommendation is to use olive oil, butter, lard, coconut oil or goose fat for frying or cooking as the fat they contain is more resistant to oxidation and produces lower levels of aldehydes and free radicals. In addition the compounds that are generated are far less damaging to our bodies.

The best advice is to eat less fried food, especially as all fried food, irrespective of what type of oil or fat it is fried in, is also very high in calories. If you do fry food minimise the amount of oil or fat that you use and drain the food well on kitchen paper before you eat it. If you do use polyunsaturated vegetable oils do not reuse them. This leads to the accumulation of aldehydes and free radicals and this makes them even more dangerous.

Our Digestive Tract

What has our digestive system got to do with the food that is making us ill? Well far more than you think.

Many scientists believe that the seeds of many health issues and chronic diseases start with our digestive tract. As a consequence it is a part of our body that is giving rise to something close to a revolution in the fields of nutrition and immunology. Hardly a week goes by without us seeing headlines on how what is often referred to as our "gut" is influencing not only our health and our ability to combat infection but also our ability to control our weight.

Strange as it may seem our intestines, especially our large intestine, contain a large diverse community of bacteria that in each of us weighs on average 1½kilos or 3½lbs. This collection of bacteria has acquired the name of the "microbiome". It is a sort of internal Eco system and it appears to be instrumental to our well being. Up until fairly recently these bacteria were more or less ignored, and it is only now that their importance is beginning to be understood. A healthy microbiome has been linked to a healthy immune system but some scientists believe that it also acts almost like a second brain with signals going from our digestive tract to our brain and not just from our brain to our digestive tract as they originally thought. The biggest influence on our microbiome is our diet and this is something that we are all able to control.

Our Gastrointestinal tract is designed to destroy the viruses and bacteria in our food before they infect our body, so it is hardly surprising that our immune system clicks rapidly into action in our digestive tract. It is now estimated that two thirds of our body's immune defenses reside there.

Our stomach uses acid to kill bacteria and other nasties that can cause disease or make us ill, but at the same time it allows beneficial bacteria which are acid tolerant to pass through into our small intestine. If your stomach is unsuccessful at getting rid of the 'bad guys' they can make their way to the small intestine and dominate your digestive tract, damaging the walls of your intestine and making you ill. Interestingly, our stomach becomes less acidic as we get older, so as we age it is less successful at getting rid of the 'bad guys'. As a consequence the number of beneficial bacteria reduces.

When we consume what is ubiquitously called 'junk food' that is laden with sugar, trans fats and polyunsaturated vegetable oils bad, unfriendly bacteria begin to flourish and good, friendly microbes begin to decline. The bad microbes produce endotoxins which our immune system detects as invaders that must be removed. The normal immune response is switched on and the start of an inflammatory cascade begins. Do other foods affect our microbiome? Well artificial sweeteners and sugar substitutes have been clearly shown to have an adverse impact on our microbiome as does a lack of fermentable fibre in our diet. Because certain types of the not so good bacterial thrive in bile and bile is needed to digest fats, the finger has also been pointed at the amount of fatty meat we consume. Too much meat, especially intensively farmed meat that has been fed on antibiotics and hormones appears to correspond to increased levels of the less desirable bacteria.

Common allergens like the casein found in milk and the gluten found in wheat can for some people be quick to spark an inflammatory cascade but stress is also a well known disrupter of our digestive system. If you have ever lost your appetite, felt sick or had bad diarrhoea before an exam or an important interview you will know what I mean.

There is evidence that stress can also inhibit the way our small intestine absorbs glucose, fructose and galactose. When this happens sugars end up making their way to the large intestine where they are fermented by the bacteria there and this can lead to discomfort and flatulence. More important though, is the fact that stress has an immediate impact on both the composition and function of the bacteria in our digestive tract and this can make the population of bacteria less diverse. When this happens the sort of bad bacteria that can cause damage begin to take over.

Given the explosion of interest in our digestive tract and microbiome it is hardly surprising that the food industry has latched onto the concept of good bugs and bad bugs. As a consequence our supermarket shelves are filling up with 'probiotic' products, products that are full of the live bacteria and yeasts that the manufacturer's claim will provide everything we need to heal our microbiome. Well, if this is possible, which foods if any will improve our microbiome? Contrary to what we are being told off the shelf probiotic drinks and yogurts are effective, but only while we are consuming them. When you stop consuming them their beneficial effect ends. More effective are traditional fermented foods like kefir, tempeh, sauerkraut and kimchee. Fermented food by its very nature is quite acidic so the bacteria it contains have had to evolve in order to survive in an acid environment. Because of this they are able to survive the acid in our stomach and make their way into our digestive tract where they can have a beneficial effect on the bacteria living there. Better still though, and a more sustainable solution, is to cut out the foods that are damaging your microbiome and in addition to fermented foods eat more prebiotic foods that support and increase the growth of good bacteria. Foods rich in indigestible fibre, in particular a prebiotic fibre called inulin that is found in onions, leeks, garlic, Jerusalem artichokes and asparagus all help to create an environment in which the good beneficial bacteria can flourish.

Inflammatory & Anti Inflammatory Foods

Many of us are unknowingly living in a body that is in a state of chronic inflammation and the biggest influence we can have on this is to change our diet.

It is clear that some foods are inflammatory because they promote and fuel inflammation, and that some foods are anti inflammatory because they calm inflammation down. So how does the food we eat during our day by day lives fit into the big picture of inflammation? How do we know which foods are inflammatory and which foods are anti-inflammatory?

As a general rule carbohydrates and meat are inflammatory. All fish, vegetables and fruit, with only a few exceptions, are anti-inflammatory. What a food contains as well as the way it is cooked affects its inflammatory potential. For instance, onions that are eaten raw are anti-inflammatory but cover them in batter and fry them in vegetable oil and they become highly inflammatory.

The type and amount of fat and Essential Fatty Acids a food contains is a key element when determining its inflammatory potential, but the vitamins, minerals and antioxidants it contains, the amount and type of carbohydrate, fibre and resistant starch, as well as other nutrients and anti-inflammatory compounds like polyphenols, all combine to create the effect the different types of food will have on our bodies. Various organisations have published 'Inflammation Factors', 'Inflammation Indexes' and 'Inflammation Ratings' using their own scoring systems, but with so many different factors coming into play it is not surprising that there is as yet no agreed 'standard' for measuring the inflammation potential of specific foods. If you look on the internet you will find sites that publish lists of how inflammatory or anti-inflammatory different foods are, but because of the different ways in which these lists have been calculated, the figures vary quite considerably. They do however give a reasonable indication of a food's inflammatory potential.

Which are the most strongly anti-inflammatory foods and which are the most strongly pro-inflammatory foods? Cold water oily fish like salmon, herring and mackerel are by far the most anti-inflammatory foods you can eat. In fact, without exception, all fish and seafood are anti-inflammatory, provided of course that it is not covered in batter or breadcrumbs and fried in vegetable oil. Surprisingly many herbs and spices like garlic, chilli, ginger and turmeric, even in small amounts, are strongly anti-inflammatory and onions, carrots, sweet potatoes, spinach, squashes and kale also come high on the list.

When it comes to the most inflammatory foods you won't be surprised to hear that it is meat and poultry, offal, sugar, refined carbohydrates, food that is fried in vegetable oil and processed foods that contain trans fats, preservative and artificial sweeteners.

At first sight the classification of some foods can be very confusing, especially as some foods contain both both pro-inflammatory and anti-inflammatory compounds. An orange for example contains large amounts of antioxidants that help reduce inflammation, but it also contains quite a large amount of the sugar fructose which can fuel inflammation. Oatmeal is another example as, like all grains, it is generally classed as being moderately inflammatory. However, there are many people who regard oatmeal as a superfood because it has low levels of fat, it is high in protein, it contains little or no gluten and it has very high levels of resistant starch, something which is lacking in our modern diet. Oatmeal also contains a fibre called beta-glucan and a powerful anti-oxidant called avenanthramide and both of these have a beneficial effect on reducing levels of so called bad cholesterol.

At the end of the day it is all about balance. If you lived on nothing but oatmeal you would not have a very good diet, but if you combine a bowl of unsweetened porridge with a chopped apple, a handful of cherries or some lightly sautéed vegetables you immediately balance out the 'inflammatory' potential of the oatmeal and give yourself a very healthy meal.

Do our bodies reflect our foods' inflammation potential? The answer to this is interesting as several 'day-by-day' and 'diary' dietary studies have shown that they do, but not to the extent that you would expect. However, when you look at large population studies the picture is completely different.

There are chemical 'markers' in our bodies that indicate how inflamed our bodies are. By measuring these markers across large populations it is clear that those of us who consume the standard 'Western Diet' have much higher levels of inflammatory markers than populations that consume a diet like the 'Mediterranean Diet'. When you look at the typical 'Western Diet' it is easy to see why. It contains large amounts of red and processed meat, dairy products, over refined carbohydrates, sugar, polyunsaturated vegetable oils and trans fats. It is low in fish, very low in fresh vegetables and fruit and sadly lacking in fibre and resistant starch. On the other hand the Mediterranean Diet is the opposite. It contains large amounts of fresh vegetables and fruit, fish and fibre. It contains moderate amounts of olive oil, which incidentally is anti-inflammatory, and red wine. It is low in red meat, processed foods, sugar, vegetable oils and trans fats.

When we look at pro and anti inflammatory foods the most important thing to remember is that inflammation is an essential part of a healthy immune response. A healthy balanced diet should provide everything we need to support it, but if you suffer from chronic inflammation you need to focus on a diet that is more anti than pro inflammatory. However, this does not mean that you have to stop eating food that promotes inflammation. Having a good balance of the right fats, proteins and carbohydrates is the key issue. Being liberal with your use of herbs and spices is a very simple way of boosting the anti-inflammatory potential of your food. Herbs and spices are close to being a 'secret weapon' when it comes to treating inflammation, especially as they are inexpensive and add an interesting dimension to our food. But, and this is a big but, they are not a wonder food. They may provide many of the trace elements, minerals and micronutrients that our body's antioxidant defense team needs, and they many have very powerful antioxidant and anti-inflammatory properties, but they cannot make a bad diet good.

Chapter Five

Eating What Is Good For Us

Are we really what we eat?

The food fibs that changed our eating habits have had a profound impact on our health and it is an impact that is definitely not for the good. Polyunsaturated vegetable oils, trans fats, sugar in all its disguises, over refined carbohydrates, brown caramelised food and a lack of vegetables and fibre in our diet are all taking their toll. We really are what we eat and diet, cooking methods and lifestyle are major factors in the dramatic increase in many of the chronic diseases that are becoming so prevalent in the Western World. This means that changes to our diet, the way we cook our food and live our daily lives will have a positive impact on our health.

Exercise

Possibly one of the biggest problems we are facing today is that with the internet and modern technology many of us are able to work, socialise and shop and hardly move a muscle. It is easy to confuse being busy with being active. The theory is that if we are using less energy we need to consume less food. Whether this is true is a matter of conjecture but one thing for certain is that very few of us are getting anywhere near enough exercise.

Regular exercise helps with insulin sensitivity and it also helps boost your immune system. Both have a positive effect in reducing oxidative stress. When you exercise your body produces some very powerful hormones; endorphins, serotonin and dopamine. At the same time the levels of stress hormones like cortisol are reduced. Endorphins are the body's natural feel good factor. When they are released through exercise they work together to make you feel good, your mood is boosted and you feel a general state of well being. You feel happy afterwards. However, do not delude yourself into thinking that you can exercise yourself out of a bad diet.

A change to your diet goes hand in hand with exercise. What sort of exercise? Well it doesn't have to be anything too strenuous, you certainly don't need to join a gym. In fact if you do not exercise regularly joining a gym is probably the last thing you should do as it can lead to " *I have got to go to the gym and work out"* syndrome that will provide a stress factor that is likely to bring with it a set of adverse consequences. Mild, gentle exercise, just ten to twenty minutes each day is all you need and it will improve your mood. Try using the stairs instead of the lift or the escalator more often. Walking is great. Just half an hour three or four times a week means that you will be getting the current recommended guideline of 150 minutes exercise a week and it will improve your health dramatically.

Where did it all go wrong?

We all lead busy lives and as a consequence quick meals and convenience foods are sometimes a necessity. For many of us cooking and preparing food is seen as a chore. Many of us would prefer to watch TV or read a book than cook. I think the problem really started when we began to 'manufacture' food, and I mean 'manufacture' in the widest sense of the word. The intensive farming of beef and poultry is just another type of manufacturing. When we started manufacturing food it became available in large quantities at a price that ordinary people could afford. At the same time it became easy for us to eat food that would otherwise take a long time to prepare and cook. Luxury foods like biscuits, cookies, cakes, chips, fries, mayonnaise and processed meats became widely available, so the ordinary man was able to eat more and at the same time adopt some of the eating habits of the rich. A hundred years ago you were lucky if you ate meat once a week. Now many people in the developed countries eat it every day, sometimes at every meal. How often do you eat chicken or turkey? Well a hundred years ago chicken and turkey were luxury foods. They were the preserve of the wealthy. The ordinary man was lucky if he ate them once a year at Christmas or Thanksgiving, now we can eat them any time we want.

How many 'manufactured' foods were available a hundred years ago? No where near the number there are today. When did they first appear on the scene? Well we know that sugar goes back a very long way. But what about breakfast cereals. They were first packaged as a wholegrain health food in the1880's but by the 1920's they began to evolve into the sugar coated flakes, hoops and puffs that we know today. Why did we change our eating habits, begin snacking between meals and adopt so much manufactured and processed foods as part of our daily diet so quickly? The answer to this would fill volumes. What we do know is that many of the manufactured foods that have come onto the scene since the early 1900's are a smoking gun when it comes to obesity, diabetes and chronic diseases and none of them are contributing positively to the health of the nation.

When it comes to the food industry, it is very difficult not to become political. However, it is an undeniable fact that food and drink manufacturing is now big business. Food and drink companies are massive international conglomerates whose only objective is to persuade us to consume more and more of their products so that they can make more and more profits for their share holders. They spend billions of dollars a year on aggressive advertising that is geared to preserving their bottom line profits and not the health and well being of the people consuming the food they make.

Manufactured foods bring with them a whole raft of problems not least of which is the addition of compounds that are designed to enhance their appearance and extend their shelf life. Most food processing takes out many of the good things and adds back in a lot of bad things. Manufactured and processed foods are generally speaking impoverished products. Because of this our diet contains too many calories that have been stripped of most of the essential trace nutrients necessary for their proper assimilation. The high-speed milling of grains like wheat results in the reduction or removal of more than twenty nutrients, including some essential fatty acids and the majority of the minerals and trace elements. In order to make your body's internally produced antioxidant team you need these minerals and trace elements. Without these antioxidants free radicals are not neutralised and oxidative stress develops at an ever-increasing rate.

Like many things in life food can be addictive and manufactured and processed foods really are addictive, the food manufacturers have made sure of that. Dietary habits are just that, habits, and like all habits they can be changed. However, urging someone to change the eating habits of a lifetime is no easy task. It is a fact that less than 20% of patients seeking medical advice are prepared to make substantial lifestyle and dietary changes. However, in the management of obesity, insulin resistance and many chronic diseases, dietary and lifestyle changes are crucially important. If your body is not functioning properly there is no magic cure or silver bullet. In order to get it back into proper working order, the essential first step towards leading a healthy life, you need a long term sustainable solution.

Over recent years we have been told that super foods and special food supplements are wonder foods that will cure all our ills. The sad reality is that you cannot rectify a diet that is overloaded with the wrong foods and completely lacking in the essential vitamins, minerals and antioxidants it so desperately needs by simply taking a one off cure. We need to look at the 'big picture' and begin eating a healthy diet, but finding out what a healthy diet is for us today not an easy matter.

For many years a major supermarket chain in the UK has been using the advertising slogan *'Every little helps'*. In their case they are saying that every penny counts towards the total amount you will save when you shop in their store. When it comes to a healthy diet every vitamin, mineral, antioxidant and micro nutrient, no matter how small, will contribute towards the well balanced diet that your body needs. If you are reading this you are one of the 20% of people who are prepared to make, or at least think about making, some major changes to your diet and lifestyle. The purpose of this book is to inform you and provide you with the information that will help you make these changes.

We each have our own individual preferences for a balance of different foods; meat and fish, fruit and vegetables, potatoes, bread, rice and pasta. Food transforms us. It provides the building blocks for the amazing body that we live in. As we age we gain weight. The average person is thought to gain around one pound a year between the age of twenty and seventy. However, it appears that calories are not quite equal when it comes to their ability to make us gain weight. Some people continue to be over weight while eating as little as 1,000 calories a day. Others stay slim even when eating four times this amount. While genetics do come into play here, it is important to remember that insulin and insulin resistance play a major part in whether or not we gain weight or lose it and inside each of us our amazing microbiome is hard at work keeping us healthy and we should not forget that this needs to be nourished and kept healthy as well.

There is no doubt that some food is good to eat, some is not quite so good and some is actually quite bad. So what are the good things that you can always eat, what are the 'not quite so good' things that you can sometimes eat or eat in moderation and what are the bad things that you should really try to avoid eating? Well the bad list is quite a challenge as it includes most of the processed and manufactured foods that have found their way into our diet over the last hundred years and many of us eat them more or less every day. So it means no more burgers, fries, chips, cookies, low fat dairy, spreads, baked goods, white bread, ice cream, fruit juice and smoothies, creamers and regular soft drinks, or at the very least cutting right back and eating them only once in a while.

ALWAYS EAT

Vegetables, pulses and whole fruit

Fish & seafood

Nuts & seeds

White, green & oolong tea

Herbs & spices

Yogurt, milk & dairy products

Eggs

Tofu, bean curd & Tempeh

Fermented foods

Butter & other saturated fats

Olives & Olive oil

Water; good old fashioned 'Adams Ale'

Whole grains & cereals

SOMETIMES EAT

Rice

Pasta

The humble potato

Meat

Chocolate and cocoa

Red wine

NEVER EAT

Polyunsaturated vegetable oils

Trans fats

Sugar & High Fructose Corn Syrup

Refined carbohydrates

Artificial sweeteners & sugar substitutes

Fruit juice & smoothies

Food that is fried, roasted & BBQ'd

Will you lose weight? Probably yes, simply because you will be eating more fibre, the amount of hidden sugar, oil and fat you eat will be significantly reduced and you will be eating modest amounts of carbohydrates and the ones you do eat will be complex. Will you feel hungry? No, because the ingredients used in the recipes in this book are packed full of flavour, fibre and nutrients that 'fill you up' and give your body the 'I don't need to eat any more' message. Eating well means that you are likely to feel healthier and you will be surprised how much energy you have.

This probably looks like quite a challenge. Put simply, the Always Sometimes Never eat diet is all about going back to basics and unless you can find a safe and reliable source of healthy manufactured food this means cooking. Can't cook, won't cook, don't know how to cook? It is not as hard as you think. After all it is only over the last fifty to sixty years that we stopped cooking. Taking back control of cooking could well be the single most important step you take on the road to eating a healthy diet. Reclaiming cooking will provide you with healthier food, it will make you self reliant and it will open a door to a more enjoyable and nourishing way of life.

Home cooked food nourishes the soul as well as they body but we need to be realistic about it. Time and energy are precious, especially during the working week so you need recipes for food that can be prepared in advance or made when you have limited time to cook, Many of the recipes in this book can also be frozen or made with ingredients from the freezer. The recipes taste good, they can be eaten by the whole family and they all have a place in a healthy diet.

Always Eat

A long list and an interesting group of food and there is more to it than meets the eye. It is all about something called Sirt Foods.

Over the last year or two a diet called The Sirt Food Diet has become one of the most talked about diets, probably because it advocates eating chocolate and drinking red wine as part of a diet. The promise is that by eating a group of foods that have been given the name of 'Sirt' foods you will switch on your skinny gene, your metabolism will change and you will burn up unwanted fat effortlessly. Whether this is true is not relevant to where Sirt Foods fit into a healthy diet, but before we can understand what Sirt Foods are and how they fit into the big picture we need some more science.

Sirt Foods are foods that enhance the action of a group of enzymes collectively known as SIRS, Silent Information Regulators, that exist inside our cells. These enzymes, which have been given the name 'sirtuins', have been the subject of intense study since they were discovered a few decades ago and some interesting discoveries have been made about the role they play in our health and well being. In lower organisms they are known to extend life span and this is probably why they initially attracted such a lot of interest. In mammals there are seven "sirt genes" each of which fulfils a different role. There is increasing evidence that the sirt genes 3 to 5 regulate ageing and age related diseases but how they do this is not yet fully understood.

What is known however, is that sirtuins play a major role in how we respond to stress and how we digest and use the food we eat. Exercise and fasting are known to 'switch them on'. When energy is in short supply, whether it is as a result of exercise or lack of food, the amount of stress inside a cell increases. The Sirtuins sense this and send out signals that change the way the cells behave. Our metabolism is geared up a notch, fat burning is switched on, our insulin response changes, inflammation is reduced, free radicals are mopped up and cells go into 'repair' mode. So rather than make new cells to replace dead or dying cells they repair the ones they have got. Simplistic, but this is the general picture, and this is where Sirtuins fit into an Always, Sometimes, Never eat diet.

In the Sirt Food Diet sirtuins are thought to help you burn up fat as well as reduce the number of fat cells you have by preventing them from duplicating. So by eating a diet high in the foods that enhance Sirtuin activity, the concept is that you lose weight. However, when it comes to eating a healthy diet there are three things that are of far greater significance than claims about weight loss.

- If you are insulin resistant or close to becoming insulin resistant, improving the way your body manages its insulin response can only be good.
- If your body is in a state of oxidative stress free radicals are over powering your body's antioxidant defences and more cells than normal are dying. So by helping your body to mop up the free radicals the sirt foods will improve the antioxidant to free radical balance and reduce this stress. Because they also change the way your cells behave by encouraging the cells go into 'repair' rather than 'destroy' mode, more cells are repaired and the number of dead cells reduces. Ultimately this leads to a general improvement in your health.
- If your body is in a state of systemic inflammation sirt foods will help reduce the inflammation.

Are Sirt foods special foods?

There is no doubt that Sirtuins play a powerful role in our health but are the foods that enhance or 'up regulate' their action special foods? The simple answer is no. Most SIRT foods form the basis of many of the healthy diets from around the world. The Mediterranean Diet and the Japanese Diet immediately come to mind and both of these diets are well known for the health and longevity of the people that consume them.

All plant based foods in the form of vegetables, fruit, tea, coffee, herbs, spices and even red wine and chocolate contain an enormous number of compounds called phytonutrients and some of these are known to directly stimulate and promote the production of Sirtuins. Unlike vitamins, phytonutrients are not essential for life. They have many powerful beneficial effects when we eat them but we can go for days, weeks and sometimes even months without them. However, the longer we go without them the more our health suffers. Over the last few decades science has identified around 25,000 different phytonutrients and it is hardly surprising that such a large group of compounds has attracted an enormous amount of interest.

Ever wondered why fruit and vegetables are so colourful? Flavonoids and carotenoids are two groups of phytonutrient compounds that give vegetables and fruit, grains, leaves and flowers their colour. Colours range from reds and orange to purple, mauve and blue. Flavonoids and carotenoids are antioxidant compounds that protect plants from being damaged by ultra violet radiation so when we eat them they provide us with antioxidants. Other phytonutrient compounds give plants scents and flavours that attract pollinators or deter predators. Anti nutrients like lectins, phytates and trypsin inhibitors are good examples of compounds that protect plants by deterring predators. Other phytonutrients protect the plant from disease so when we eat them they provide us with compounds that have anti inflammatory, anti bacterial and anti fungal properties. Some phytonutrients are known to help reduce blood pressure and so called bad LDL cholesterol and some are thought to be able to protect us from developing cancers.

When it comes to their ability to stimulate the production of Sirtuins not all plants are created equal. As a general rule the darker the leafy vegetable or the brighter the colour the more powerful they are, so it is hardly surprising that kale, spinach, chard, broccoli, cabbage, carrots, onions, sweet potatoes, peas, beans, squash, egg plants, peppers, pumpkin, tomatoes, black currents, blue berries and red berries like strawberries and raspberries are at the top of the list of SIRT foods. But all vegetables and fruit, without exception, bring with them a host of health benefits and there is plenty of scientific evidence to support this.

Man as a species is an omnivore and our digestive tract is that of an omnivore. For hundreds and thousands of years seasonal vegetables, pulses and fruit combined with modest amounts of meat, fish and complex carbohydrates were our staple diet. Now for many of us vegetables have fallen off the menu and for some they have vanished completely. Whether or not The Sirt Food diet is a fad diet when it comes to losing weight remains to be seen, but if it leaves a legacy of healthier eating with vegetables and fruit once again the core elements of our diet then it can only be a good thing.

Vegetables, Pulses & Fruit

Why?

Vegetables and fruit are simply packed full of goodness and they taste great. They contain vitamins, minerals, trace elements, large amounts of antioxidants and fibre. Most vegetables are alkaline and many have antioxidant and anti-inflammatory properties. Polyphenols, flavonoids, anthocyanins, carotenoids, quercetin, resveratrol are just some of a long list of health giving compounds that fruit and vegetables contain. You name it they've got it and because they are so colourful they look wonderful on your plate.

Green leafy vegetables, celery, beans, sweet potatoes, winter squashes, peppers, aubergines or eggplants, pumpkins, berries, apples, oranges, lemons and limes. The list of vegetables and fruit that are available for us to eat is massive. We are wired to eat them and whether you eat them raw or cooked, they form an essential part of a healthy diet. At least five portions of vegetables and fruit a day is really good advice.

Should you be concerned about fruits that contain a lot of fructose? Is it possible to eat too much fruit? Guidelines vary from a minimum of two portions a day to four or more, but there is increasing evidence that low doses of fructose from whole natural fruit may actually benefit the control of blood sugar. In reality unless you eat your way through several hundred grams of grapes or an awful lot of apples you are unlikely to be eating enough during a day to cause any real problems in terms of excess fructose consumption as the fibre in the fruit will slow down the rate at which it is absorbed.

It is interesting that one of the fruits often labelled as 'never eat' are bananas. Pop ups to this effect frequently appear when you do an internet search. The reason for this is that ripe bananas contain quite a lot of carbohydrate. A medium size banana weighing 120 gram contains just over 100 kcal and about 25 gram of carbohydrate in the form of sugar. Is this sufficient reason to not eat bananas? Well the answer is no. Like most fruit bananas are healthy and nutritious. They contain fibre, potassium, magnesium, vitamin C, vitamin B6, copper, manganese and iodine. The less ripe the banana is the better it is to eat. Unripe bananas contain large amounts of resistant starch and pectin. As well as making you feel full and slowing down the rate at which the sugar in the banana is absorbed, both of these act as prebiotics and provide a healthy environment for the bacteria in your digestive tract to flourish. As the banana ripens this resistant starch is converted into sugar. The riper the banana the more sugar it contains, so the basic rule is to eat your bananas as under ripe as possible.

One group of vegetables that is often overlooked are salad leaves. Many of us regard them as a 'garnish' that is rarely eaten. However, the reality is that when you take into account their calorie and fibre content salad leaves are one of the most nutritious group of vegetables available to us. The darker and redder the leaves the more beneficial compounds they contain, and when you eat them with dressings made from olive oil and lemon juice or oily fruits like avocado you absorb even more of these compounds. One other thing that is interesting to note is that studies have consistently shown that when they eat salad leaves before or as part of a meal people actually eat less.

Pulses

With the exception of baked beans very few of us eat pulses. This is a pity as pulses are a cheap source of protein, fibre, vitamins, minerals and resistant starch and they also count towards your 'five a day'. As well as being a highly nutritious vegetable that is low in carbohydrate the fibre in them is thought to help reduce the risk of developing heart disease and type 2 diabetes. Pulses come in the form of beans, peas and lentils. All of these are edible seeds that grow in pods so, like grains and cereals, they contain anti nutrients and some of these need to be removed by cooking. With the exception of lentils and fava beans, all pulses need to be boiled for at least ten minutes before being left to simmer slowly until they are cooked.

Pulses are the staple food of millions of people around the world; red beans, turtle beans, navy beans, chick peas, butter beans, borlotti beans, haricot beans, red and green lentils, fava beans, mung beans, adzuki beans and dried split peas are just some of them. Most uncooked pulses contain between 20% and 25% protein by weight. This is double that of wheat and more than three times that of rice. On average a 175 gram cooked serving of pulses contains around 10 gram of protein and between 5 and 10 grams of fibre. For vegetarians and vegans pulses are a primary source of protein but for meat eaters trying to reduce the amount of meat they consume they provide a valuable addition to casseroles and stews.

Like bananas pulses are a valuable source of prebiotic fibre that feeds the healthy bacteria in your microbiome, slows down your digestion and helps make you feel full for longer. This fibre is renowned for the effect pulses have on your bowel as it increases the amount of gas produced. For most people this is a temporary problem. If you have never eaten pulses before most nutritionists recommend that you begin with small portions and gradually increase the portion size in line with how comfortable you feel.

How?

Eat as many vegetables and as much fruit as you want. They are on 'free issue'. Where possible eat fruit and vegetables unpeeled. We need to remember that the phytonutrients in food exist first and foremost to protect the food itself from damage. So the whole food, often including its skin, is often more powerful than individual isolated elements.

Substitute beans and pulses for potatoes, rice and pasta. Why? Because 100 grams of red beans contains 8 grams of complex carbohydrate, which is much less than the 80 grams of starchy carbohydrate in the same amount of rice, potatoes or pasta and they are also a valuable source of protein and fibre. Puréed and mixed with herbs, ground nuts and yogurt, vegetables make great dips and spreads. Instead of crisps and chips try snacking on celery and sticks of carrot, cucumber and sliced red and green peppers.

Our palettes vary enormously and to some people green vegetables can have an unpleasant 'sulphur' taste. Adding a small amount of chopped basil or basil pesto after they are cooked is an effective way of masking the sulphur taste. This is a good trick when you are encouraging young children to eat vegetables and it often works.

Should we eat our vegetables raw or cooked?

We are often told that raw vegetables are more nutritious than cooked ones but this is not necessarily the case. Cooking vegetables, and in particular pulses, can have the benefit of neutralising anti-nutrient enzymes that interfere with the assimilation of minerals and trace elements. At the same time it also breaks down the cells in the vegetable and this makes it easier for us to digest and absorb the nutrients the vegetables contain. Carrots and tomatoes are good examples of how cooking can increase the nutritional content. The intense vibrant colour of these vegetables comes from a very powerful antioxidant called lycopene. With some vegetables cooking can damage some of their nutritional content but when tomatoes and carrots are cooked the lycopene in them actually becomes more available and easier to assimilate. This makes them a very valuable and powerful source of antioxidants. One other benefit of cooking is that it has the effect of reducing the volume of a vegetable and this makes it easier for us to eat more and obtain more beneficial phytonutrients. Most of us would baulk at the idea of eating a whole bag of spinach but steamed or lightly sautéed the spinach rapidly shrinks to an acceptable volume.

At the opposite end of the spectrum when some foods are cooked, especially when they are boiled, some of the phytonutrients are leached out into the cooking water and lost. Broccoli is a good example of this as boiling can destroy between 20% and 30% of its vitamin C. On the other hand steaming it or cooking it in a microwave reduces the vitamin C only by 10%. The general message is whether you eat your vegetables raw, steamed, microwaved or lightly sautéed depends as much on your personal preference as the vegetable itself. However, unless you are going to use the cooking water for soup avoid boiling them.

Should we keep our fruit and vegetables in the fridge?

Like cooking this depends entirely on the fruit or vegetable. Some are better left out on the kitchen work top to continue to ripen and develop more phytonutrients while others are better stored in the fridge. The bottom line is that leaving fruit out of the fridge at ambient temperature will speed up the rotting as well as the ripening process. If you are able to shop and buy your fruit and vegetables frequently then this will not be a problem but if you only shop once a week, keeping your fruit and vegetables in the fridge would probably be the most practical.

Roasted Tomato, Feta & Lentil Salad

PUY LENTILS ARE A USEFUL STORE CUPBOARD INGREDIENT AND THEY DO NOT NEED TO BE SOAKED BEFORE THEY ARE COOKED.

SERVES 4

100g/3½oz Puy lentils
300ml/10 fl oz (½pt) water
12 medium size tomatoes cut in half
1 tbsp balsamic vinegar
1 tsp sea salt flakes
6 spring onions sliced
200g/7oz feta OR 4 hard boiled eggs cut into quarters
2 punnets of mustard cress
large handful of basil leaves, roughly chopped
Juice ½ lemon

Pre heat the oven to 200°C/ 400°F/Gas 5

Wash and drain the lentils and put them into a saucepan with the water. Bring them to the boil, cover and reduce the heat to low. Simmer them for 40 to 45 minutes until they are tender. Drain off any liquid that is left.

Put the tomatoes cut side up onto a baking tray lined with non stick foil. Sprinkle over the salt and drizzle over the balsamic vinegar. Roast the tomatoes for 30 minutes.

Put the lentils into a large bowl and stir in the lemon juice. Add the tomatoes, sliced spring onions, chopped basil and the mustard cress. Divide between 4 plates and scatter over the crumbled feta or boiled egg

Banana Blue Berry Muffins

YOU CAN USE FRESH OR FROZEN FRUIT TO MAKE THESE. USE BLUE BERRIES OR BLACK CURRENTS. THE RECIPE MAKES 12 50ML/2 FL OZ MUFFINS.

Makes 12

125g/4½oz wholegrain spelt
100g/3½oz ground almonds
1 large free range egg
3 tbsp olive oil
1 heaped tbsp dark unrefined Muscavado sugar
2 bananas weighing about 300g/10½oz
1 tsp baking powder
1 tsp bicarbonate of soda
85g/3oz blue berries or black currents
1 tbsp demerera sugar (optional)

Pre heat the oven to 180°C/ 350°F/Gas 4 and grease the muffin tins.

Mix together the spelt, ground almonds, sugar, baking powder and bicarbonate of soda. You may need to break up the lumps in the sugar with your fingers.

Put the bananas, egg and oil into a bowl and whiz it with a hand blender until you have a smooth cream.

Add the dry ingredients and mix well. Fold in the blue berries or black currents and spoon into the muffin tins. If you are using it, sprinkle the demerera sugar on top and bake for 20 minutes.

Stuffed Mushrooms

LARGE FLAT MUSHROOMS ARE GREAT FOR STUFFING WITH A WIDE RANGE OF DIFFERENT FILLINGS. THESE ARE STUFFED WITH A SPICY WALNUT SALSA MIXED WITH RED BEANS, SPINACH AND AUBERGINE. YOU CAN TOP THE STUFFED MUSHROOMS WITH CRUMBLED FETA OR GRILLED GOATS CHEESE. THE STUFFING MAKES AN EXCELLENT SALAD WHEN SERVED ON ITS OWN.

SERVES 4

4 large flat Portabella (Crimini) mushrooms with stalks removed
2 tbsp olive oil
1 tsp chilli flakes
500g/1lb 2oz frozen spinach
1 aubergine cut into 1cm/½in pieces
400g/14 oz can red kidney beans, drained and rinsed
85g/ 3oz chopped walnuts or pecan nuts
2 tbsp Worcestershire sauce
2 tbsp cider vinegar
1 clove garlic crushed
1 tsp Sambol Oelek or finely chopped red chilli
2 tsp walnut oil
1 tbsp chopped parsley
2 tbsp chopped coriander

Pre heat the oven to 200°C/ 400°F/Gas 5.

Wipe the mushrooms and put them onto a dish that is large enough to hold them in a singe layer. Alternatively put them on a baking tray lined with foil. Mix together the olive oil and chilli flakes and drizzle this over the mushrooms. Cover with foil and bake for 20 minutes.

Cook the frozen spinach in line with the instructions on the package and when it is cool enough to handle squeeze out as much moisture as possible.

Chop up the mushrooms stalks and put them with the aubergine into a microwave bowl. Cover and cook on full power for 5 minutes.

To make the salsa, mix together the walnuts, the Worcestershire sauce, the vinegar, walnut oil, garlic, Sambol Oelek, the chopped parsley and the coriander.

Mix together the red beans, walnut salsa, cooked aubergine and spinach. Drain into this the juices from the cooked mushrooms. Spoon this bean mixture into the mushrooms, cover with foil and bake for 10 minutes.

If you are using the crumbled feta put is on top of the mushrooms and serve. If you are using the goats cheese pre heat the grill, put the goats cheese on top of the mushrooms and grill until the cheese begins to turn lightly brown. Serve immediately.

Spinach & Red Pepper Moussaka

THIS IS A CROSS BETWEEN A SPINACH PIE AND A MOUSSAKA. TRADITIONALLY A SPINACH PIE IS COOKED IN A CASE OF FILO PASTRY AND A MOUSSAKA IS MADE WITH A MEAT STEW THAT IS COOKED BETWEEN LAYERS OF AUBERGINE. LIKE MOST AUBERGINE DISHES THIS MOUSSAKA FREEZES WELL SO YOU CAN FREEZE ANY LEFTOVERS OR MAKE IT IN ADVANCE ESPECIALLY FOR THE FREEZER. IF YOU DO FREEZE IT YOU DO NOT NEED TO COMPLETE THE FINAL BAKING PROCESS. YOU CAN USE FRESH PEPPERS THAT YOU ROAST YOURSELF OR YOU CAN USE READY ROASTED PEPPERS THAT ARE SOLD IN JARS AND CANS.

SERVES 4

600g/1lb 5oz aubergine plus olive oil for brushing

400g /14 oz cooked spinach or Swiss chard

2 tbsp pine nuts lightly toasted

200g /7 oz feta crumbled

6 spring onions finely sliced

3 large red peppers OR a jar of roasted red peppers

For the béchamel sauce

40g / 1½oz plain flour

500ml / 18 fl oz milk

60g / 2oz grated parmesan

1 egg beaten

Grated nutmeg and ground black pepper

Preheat the oven to 180°C/ 350°F/Gas 4 and Grease a large dish, about 5cm/2 inches deep.

Slice the aubergines into rounds 1cm /½ inch thick. Line two baking trays with foil and brush them with oil. Put the sliced aubergines onto the trays and lightly brush them with oil. Bake them at 180°C for 15 minutes. The aubergine should be soft but not brown. Put the cooked aubergine to one side

If you are using fresh red peppers, turn the oven up to 200°C/ 400°F/Gas 5. Cut the red peppers in quarters and roast them for 30 minutes until the skin is beginning to blister and look charred. Put them into a dish, cover them with cling film and leave them to cool a little. Peel the skins off of the peppers and tear them into strips. Reserve any oil that has come out of them.

Make the béchamel sauce. Melt the butter on a gentle heat and stir in the flour. Cook gently for a couple of minutes. You do not want the flour to take on any colour.

Using a whisk, slowly add the milk and keep whisking. Most recipes tell you to warm the milk when making a sauce to prevent lumps forming. If you use a whisk there is no need to warm the milk. When all the milk is added stir in the grated parmesan and cook gently for 5 minutes, stirring occasionally. Turn off the heat.

Squeeze the spinach or chard to make sure it is dry and mix it with the toasted pine nuts, chopped spring onions and the crumbled feta.

Pour about a quarter of the béchamel sauce over the bottom of the dish and place a layer of the cooked aubergine on top. Add the spinach mixture and on top of this pour another quarter of the béchamel sauce.

Put in another layer of cooked aubergine and then the red peppers. Top the peppers with the remaining aubergine.

Beat the egg and mix it with the remaining béchamel sauce and pour this over the top layer of aubergine.

Bake for 45 minutes. Serve with a green salad or some green vegetables.

French Bean, Roquefort & Nut Salad
YOU CAN USE PECAN NUTS OR WALNUTS AND ANY TYPE OF BLUE CHEESE TO MAKE THIS.

SERVES 4
300g/10½oz fine French beans
150g/5½oz Roquefort or other blue cheese broken into small pieces
100g/3½oz pecan nuts or walnuts roughly chopped
1 large or 2 small baby gem lettuce
3 tbsp olive oil
1 tbsp Balsamic vinegar

Cook the French beans in boiling water for 3 minutes until they are just tender. Drain and rinse them in cold water.

Wash and dry the lettuce and cut it into pieces lengthways.

Put the olive oil and balsamic vinegar into a jar and give it a shake.

Mix the lettuce, French beans and walnuts together and sprinkle over the cheese. Cover and refrigerate.

Just before serving stir in a half of the dressing. Serve the rest of the dressing in a separate bowl.

Beans in Red Mole Sauce with Avocado Salsa

THIS IS A TASTE OF MEXICO AT ITS BEST AND YES, IT REALLY DOES CONTAIN COCOA. AS THE SAUCE FREEZES WELL IT IS WORTH MAKING A BATCH FOR THE FREEZER. IF YOU DO DECIDE TO FREEZE IT LEAVE OUT THE GARLIC AS THIS CAN SOMETIME GIVE RISE TO A SLIGHTLY MUSTY FLAVOUR. YOU CAN ADD ANY TYPE OF BEAN OR VEGETABLE TO THE SAUCE AND IT ALSO WORKS WELL WITH FIRM TOFU OR TEMPEH AND THE MICRO PROTEIN QUORN.

SERVES 6
FOR THE SAUCE
2 tbsp olive oil
1 large red onion finely chopped
3 cloves garlic crushed
3 tbsp cocoa powder
1 tsp chilli powder
2 tsp ground cumin
1 tsp smoked paprika
1 tbsp sweet paprika
½ tsp salt
1 tbsp dried oregano
2 x 400g/14oz cans chopped tomatoes
2 red peppers finely sliced or diced
400g/14 oz can red or black beans
400g/14 oz black eyed beans
AVOCADO SALSA
4 tbsp finely chopped fresh coriander
1 large avocado
Juice of half a lemon or a whole lime
1 tbsp finely chopped red onion
Natural unsweetened Greek style
yoghurt to serve

Reserve a small hand full of the red peppers for a garnish. Heat the olive oil in a large saucepan. Add the onion, garlic and the rest of the red peppers and sauté over a medium heat for 5 to 10 minutes. Do not let the onion or garlic brown.

Mix together the cocoa powder, chilli, cumin, both types of paprika, salt and oregano. Add this to the onion and pepper mixture, stir well and cook, stirring all the time, for a minute or two to bring out the flavour of the spices.

Add the canned tomatoes. Give everything a good stir, bring to the boil, turn down the heat and simmer gently for 10 minutes.

Pre heat the oven to 160°C/ 325°F/Gas 3

Drain and rinse the beans and add them to the sauce. Bring everything back to the boil, then turn off the heat and transfer the beans and sauce to an oven proof dish or casserole. Cook for 30 – 40 minutes while you prepare the salsa.

TO MAKE THE AVOCADO SALSA

Cut the avocado in half. Remove the stone using a small spoon, then peel and chop the avocado into small pieces. Stir in the lemon juice and add the finely chopped red onion and the chopped coriander.

Serve the beans garnished with the reserved red peppers and with the natural yoghurt and the avocado salsa in separate bowls.

Tfaya with Chickpeas

TFAYA IS A DISH OF STEWED ONIONS THAT IS EATEN THROUGHOUT NORTH AFRICA AND THE MIDDLE EAST. IT IS USUALLY SERVED AS AN ACCOMPANIMENT TO MEAT DISHES BUT IT WORKS REALLY WELL WITH NUT LOAFS, FIRM TOFU AND TEMPEH, CHICKPEAS AND OTHER TYPES OF BEANS. IT CAN BE KEPT IN THE FRIDGE FOR A DAY OR TWO AND IT FREEZES REALLY WELL. SERVE THE TFAYA WITH A SELECTION OF GREEN VEGETABLES OR A SALAD.

SERVES 4

1Kg/2 lb 4oz white onions finely sliced
50g/1¾oz raisins
3 tbsp butter or ghee
1 tsp ground black pepper
1 tsp ground cinnamon
1 tsp ground ginger
½ tsp turmeric
Large pinch saffron strands
2 tbsp honey
125ml/4 fl oz water
2 tsp vegetable stock powder
Finely grated zest of half a small lemon
juice of 1 lemon
2 preserved lemons de-seeded and finely chopped
400g/14oz can chickpeas, drained and rinsed

The onions in this recipe need long slow cooking so if you use a non stick saucepan if you have one.

Put the saffron strands into a cup or jug and add 125ml/4 fl oz boiling water and the vegetable stock powder.

Heat the butter in a saucepan over a medium heat and add the onions. Stir them and cook for 5 minutes.

Add the pepper, ginger, cinnamon, turmeric, lemon zest and salt. Give everything a good stir and add the saffron stock, raisins and the honey. Bring to the boil, cover, reduce the heat and simmer very slowly for 45 minutes. Check the onions a couple of times to make sure they are not sticking.

This is where we move into the 'naughty but nice' stage of this recipe as the onions now need to be caramelised. Take the lid off of the saucepan, increase the heat and cook the onions, stirring all the time until most of the fluid has evaporated and some of them begin to look slightly brown. Be careful as you do not want the onions to burn. Take them off the heat, add the lemon juice and preserved lemon and put the lid back on the saucepan.

When you are ready to serve the Tfaya put the chickpeas into a microwave bowl, cover and cook them following the instructions on the tin. When they are cooked stir them into the onion mixture.

Carrot, Mango & Coriander Salad

A STRANGE MIXTURE OF INGREDIENTS, BUT THIS SALAD TASTES ABSOLUTELY DELICIOUS. IT GOES EXTREMELY WELL WITH FISH, ESPECIALLY SALMON, TROUT AND SMOKED MACKEREL. YOU CAN SERVE THE SALAD ON ITS OWN OR ADD CHICKPEAS OR BEANS TO MAKE IT INTO A SUBSTANTIAL MEAL. UNFORTUNATELY ITS PREPARATION IS SOMEWHAT LABOUR INTENSIVE AS IT INVOLVES A LOT OF PEELING AND SLICING. IF YOU CAN OBTAIN ONE OF THE SOUR GREEN MANGOS THAT ARE GROWN ESPECIALLY FOR SAVOURY DISHES ALL THE BETTER. OTHERWISE USE THE MOST UNDER RIPE MANGO YOU CAN FIND.

SERVES 4

1 very large green under ripe mango
350g/12oz carrots
1 small red onion peeled and finely chopped
3 - 4 tbsp finely chopped coriander OR
30g/1oz ready made coriander pesto
Grated zest of 1 lime
Juice of 1 lime
1 tsp Sambol Oelek or chilli paste
1tbsp rice vinegar
1 tbsp Thai fish sauce
1 preserved lemon
3 tbsp lightly toasted cashew nuts and pumpkin seeds

First make the salad dressing by mixing together the zest and juice of a lime, the Sambol Oelek (you can use more than 1 tsp if you like your food spicy), the rice vinegar, the Thai fish sauce and the chopped coriander or pesto.

Peel the carrots and slice them very thinly along their length. Then cut each long slice into narrow very thin mandolin strips.

Boil some water in a saucepan and blanch the carrots for 2 minutes. Drain and refresh them in cold water.

Cut the stone from the mango. Peel the halves of mango and slice the flesh into thin slices. Now cut each of these thin slices into narrow mandolin strips. Put them into a large bowl and pour on the dressing.

Drain the carrots and add the them to the mango in the bowl and give everything a good stir.

Stir in the finely chopped red onion. You can use spring onions if you prefer but the red onion gives the salad a better colour and more intense flavour.

Cut the preserved lemon in half, take out the pips and cut it into very small pieces. Stir it into the salad.

Lastly add the toasted seeds. You can use more or less toasted seeds according to taste. Cover and leave the salad for at least half an hour for the flavours to develop.

The salad will keep for up to two days if stored in the fridge but the longer you keep it the more the texture will reduce.

Chinese Leaf, Red Pepper & Sweetcorn Salad

CHINESE LEAF IS A VALUABLE STORE CUPBOARD INGREDIENT AS IT IS AVAILABLE ALL THE YEAR ROUND AND IT KEEPS WELL. THIS IS A BRIGHT, COLOURFUL SALAD THAT WILL KEEP FOR 2 DAYS IN A COVERED CONTAINER IN THE FRIDGE. SERVE IT ON ITS OWN OR WITH A DRESSING OF YOUR CHOICE.

SERVES 4 - 6

1 large sweet Ramiro pepper
325g/11 ½oz can sweetcorn kernels
4 spring onions finely sliced
½ Chinese Leaf Cabbage
2 punnets of mustard cress

Remove the seeds from the red pepper and cut it into thin rings. Finely shred the Chinese Leaf.

Rinse and drain the sweetcorn kernels, put them into a large bowl and mix them with the mustard cress.

Stir in the red pepper and Chinese Leaf and the spring onions.

Tuscan Fish & Bean Salad

THIS IS A FAMOUS DISH FROM TUSCANY THAT IS ONE OF THOSE 'INSTANT' OUT OF THE STORE CUPBOARD MEALS. YOU WILL NEED GOOD QUALITY TUNA.

SERVES 2 - 4

400g/14oz borlotti or cannellini beans drained and rinsed
120g/4¼ oz can 'no drain' tuna steak in spring water
3 spring onions cut into match stick size slices
Salt and pepper to taste
2 tbsp lemon juice
2 tbsp olive oil
1 tbsp finely chopped parsley or chervil.
50g/1¾oz cooked fine French Beans
30g/1oz baby spinach leaves

Put the olive oil and lemon juice together in a jar and give it a good shake.

Mix the borlotti beans, spring onions and the French Beans together in a bowl and stir in the dressing.

Break the tuna into small pieces and arrange them on top of the beans. Scatter the parsley or chervil on top and serve on a bed of baby spinach leaves.

Tomato & Lentil Soup

EASY AND QUICK TO MAKE, THIS IS A BASIC SOUP THAT YOU CAN TRANSFORM INTO SOMETHING COMPLETELY DIFFERENT BY SIMPLY CHANGING THE HERBS AND SPICES YOU USE. YOU CAN ALSO 'DRESS IT UP' BY DRIZZLING OVER FLAVOURED OILS AND SPRINKLING ON CHOPPED HERBS, TOASTED NUTS AND SEEDS.

SERVES 4

400g/14oz tin chopped tomatoes
3 tbsp tomato purée
1 large red onion roughly chopped
1 stick celery roughly chopped
1 large carrot roughly chopped
100g/3½oz red lentils
1 tbsp olive oil
1 tsp Sambol Oelek or ½ tsp chilli powder (optional)
700ml/25 fl oz/1¼pt vegetable stock
3 cloves of garlic roughly chopped
4 tbsp natural unsweetened Greek style yoghurt
Handful of torn basil or oregano leaves
1 tsp ready made basil pesto mixed with 2 tbsp olive oil (optional)
1 tbsp toasted pine nuts

Wash and pick over the red lentils and make sure that there is no grit in them. Leave them to drain while you prepare the vegetables.

Heat the olive oil and lightly sauté the onion, garlic, celery and carrot for 3 or 4 minutes. Don't let them brown. Add the tin of chopped tomatoes, the tomato purée, the Sambol Oelek and chilli.

Add the vegetable stock and the lentils. Give everything a good stir, bring it to the boil, cover and simmer for 30 - 40 minutes until the lentils are tender.

Using a hand blender blend the soup until it is smooth. Stir in the yoghurt and the torn basil leaves. If you are using the basil pesto and olive oil, drizzle it over the soup just before serving and sprinkle n the toasted pine nuts.

VARIATIONS:

For a Middle Eastern flavour omit the yoghurt and basil and add 1 tsp ground cumin, 1 tsp dried dill and ½ tsp ground cardamom seeds when you add the tin of tomatoes, add the Sambol Oelek or chilli powder with ½ tsp smoked paprika,1 tsp sweet paprika, 2 tsp ground cumin, 2 heaped tsp dried oregano when you add the tin of tomatoes. Garnish with chopped coriander

For an Indian twist omit the yoghurt and basil, make sure you add the Sambol Oelek or chilli powder and add 2 tbsp grated ginger, 2 tsp ground coriander, 1 tsp ground cumin, ½ tsp turmeric, ½ tsp ground fenugreek and the grated zest of a lime when you add the tin of tomatoes. Squeeze over the juice of the lime just before serving

Onion Soup

THIS SOUP IS A REALLY SIMPLE SOUP TO MAKE. THE DRY VERMOUTH AND GRATED RAW ONION ADDED AT THE END GIVE IT AN EXTRA SPECIAL TWIST. IF YOU HAVE SOME TRUFFLE OIL JUST A SMALL AMOUNT SPRINKLED ON WHEN THE SOUP IS SERVED TASTES AMAZING.

SERVES 4

700g/1 lb 9 oz onions peeled and thinly sliced
2 tbsp grated onion
400g/14oz potatoes peeled and sliced
3 tbsp olive oil
1.7Lt/3pt vegetable stock
4 tbsp dry vermouth (optional)
4 tbsp fromage frais or natural unsweetened yoghurt
¼ tsp grated nutmeg
salt and pepper to taste
4 tbsp grated parmesan to serve OR some truffle oil

Heat the olive oil in a large saucepan and add the sliced onions and the potato. Sauté them for 5 minutes and then add the stock. Bring to the boil, cover, reduce the heat and simmer them for 20 minutes until the potatoes and onions are tender

Use a hand blender to blend the soup until it is smooth. Add the dry vermouth and season to taste with the grated nutmeg, salt and black pepper.

When you are ready to serve the soup stir in the grated onion and fromage frais and drizzle on the truffle oil if you are using it. Serve the grated Parmesan in a separate bowl.

Red Bean Burgers with Guacamole

THESE BURGERS ARE QUICK AND EASY TO MAKE AND THEY FREEZE WELL. THE RECIPE FOR THE TOASTED OATMEAL COATING IS IN THE GRAINS AND CEREALS SECTION.

SERVES 4
FOR THE BURGERS

200g/7oz finely chopped red onion
200g/7oz red cabbage finely sliced
2 x 400g/14 oz cans red kidney beans, drained and rinsed
175g/6oz firm tofu
2 tbsp olive oil
2 tsp ground cumin
2 tsp smoked paprika
2 tbsp sweet paprika
1 tsp chilli powder
4 tbsp chopped coriander
150g/5½oz cooked millet
Toasted oatmeal coating

Heat the oil in a saucepan and fry the red onion and the red cabbage for a few minutes. Keep stirring to prevent the cabbage from sticking. Turn down the heat to low and add the ground cumin, the smoked paprika, the sweet paprika and the chilli power. Give everything a quick stir and then add about 3 tbsp water. Cover the pan and cook for 20 minutes. Stir it occasionally to make sure it is not sticking. Leave the onion and cabbage to cool for about half an hour.

Put the tofu with half of the red beans and half of the onion and cabbage mixture into a bowl and blitz them with a hand blender until you have a slightly chunky paste.

GUACAMOLE

2 to 3 fresh chillies finely chopped OR 2
tsp Sambol Oelek
2 medium tomatoes finely chopped
1 tbsp finely chopped onion
1 clove garlic crushed
2 tbsp chopped fresh coriander
2 large or 3 medium ripe avocados
Lemon or lime juice to taste

Add the rest of the red beans, the rest of the onion and cabbage mixture and the chopped coriander. Blend lightly. You want to have the burgers blended enough for everything to stick together. You want some whole beans and pieces of cabbage. You don't want to turn it into a mush. Stir in the cooked millet and leave the mixture to cool for an hour or two before moving on to the next stage.

Put some fine polenta or toasted oatmeal coating onto a plate. Flour your hands with it, take a large heaped tablespoon of the mixture and form it into a burger shapes about 7cm/3in in diameter. Put the burgers onto a tray lined with cling film or non stick foil and put them into the fridge until you cook them. At this stage you can also freeze them.

To cook the burgers, oil a large non stick pan and fry them for 5 minutes on each side until a crust forms. Alternatively, lightly brush them with oil, put them onto a non stick baking tray and bake them at 200°C/ 400°F/Gas 5 for 15 to 20 minutes.

TO MAKE THE GUACAMOLE

Peel and mash the avocado and mix it with the other ingredients.

Add 1 or 2 tablespoons of lemon juice and mix well. Leave the stone in the guacamole until you are ready to eat it as for some reason this slows down the oxidation process. Do not refrigerate. If you do the guacamole will go brown.

.

Fish & Seafood

Why?

Fish is an excellent source of protein and other vital nutrients like selenium, zinc and iron. It also contains large amounts of Omega 3 Essential Fatty Acids in the easily assimilated form of EPA, eicosapentaenoic acid, and DHA, decosahexaenoic acid. These are both known to be good for your heart, your brain and even your mood. Most people do not consume enough Omega 3 fatty acids and diets that are low in them have been consistently linked to cardio vascular disease. Cold water oily fish like salmon, sardines, herring, mackerel, trout, and halibut are all excellent sources of Omega-3 but all fish, including shellfish and white fish are a good choice as part of a healthy diet. It is a well recognised fact that people who eat a diet that contains large amounts of fish and sea food live longer and healthier lives and there is emerging evidence that it is the Omega 3 in the fish oils that help slow the ageing process.

Like meat, some of the fish we eat today is farmed and this gives rise to ethical as well as health issues. Salmon in particular is something of a hot topic when it comes to fish farming and this is important as it is a fish that has the highest amounts of Omega 3 Essential Fatty Acids. Salmon is now the biggest selling fish in the UK with sales of £700 million in 2014. With stocks of wild salmon falling rapidly, half of the salmon sold worldwide now comes from fish farms. At first farming salmon seemed like a positive step towards reducing the pressure on wild fish stocks, but this optimism was quickly overtaken by concerns about the salmon farming industry's reliance on artificial feeds and the use of chemicals to treat sea lice. As a result farmed salmon has now acquired something of a bad reputation. Farmed salmon is fed on high fat artificial feed and this means that farmed salmon has three times the fat of wild salmon. The problem with this increased amount of fat is that instead of it being in the ratio of ten Omega 3 to one Omega 6 as found in wild salmon, the fat in the farmed salmon is in the ratio of between three and four Omega 3 to each Omega 6. While this ratio is not ideal it is still the right way round, three or four times more Omega 3 than Omega 6 and this makes it a healthy food to eat.

On one hand we are being told to eat more fish because its good for us and on the other we are being told that we should not be eating it because it is high in mercury and other things that are bad for us. Should you be worried about mercury in fish? Because it is exposed to environmental pollution all fish and shellfish contains mercury. Some types of fish contain only trace amounts while others contain much more.

Mercury is a problem because it deactivates some of the enzymes in our bodies that are dependent on selenium and these enzymes are extremely important, especially when it comes to our brain. However, in addition to mercury fish and seafood contains selenium and while we are given dire warnings about the dangers of mercury, what we are not told is that provided the fish we eat contains more selenium than mercury there is no danger. With the exception of pilot whale, shark, tilefish, swordfish and king mackerel, fish contains more selenium than mercury, so cod, salmon, haddock, herring and sardines are perfectly safe to eat. It is interesting to note that according to the US National Fisheries Institute there has never been a confirmed case of mercury poisoning in the United States that was caused by eating fish or seafood.

We are all getting mixed messages about eating fish, but irrespective of whether it is wild or farmed eating fish leads to a massive improvement in our intake of Omega 3 fatty acids, something that is in very short supply in our modern Western diet. When you compare the 1,000mg of Omega 3 a 125 gram portion of oily fish contains to the 35mg found in the same amount of lean grass fed beef, it is clear to see how important fish is in a healthy diet.

How?

Substitute fish for meat in your diet and in line with the FDA and American Heart Association try to eat it at least two times a week. Now, unless you live near the coast or have access to a good fishmonger, fresh fish is not so easy to obtain. Trout and salmon can usually be found but other than this you will probably have to buy frozen fish. Just remember to thaw it slowly and then wash and dry it thoroughly in order to remove any oils that have oxidised. Unfortunately oily fish like sardines, herring and mackerel do not freeze well so you may have to resort to tins. Just make sure the fish is tinned in water or olive oil and not sunflower oil as the sunflower oil transforms the fish from a healthy option to a very unhealthy one. One way the northern Europeans preserve their oily fish, especially herring, is to pickle them. Bismark herrings and roll mops are usually sold in jars and as they require no cooking they are quick and easy to prepare. Despite the fact that they are salted and then preserved in vinegar that is sometimes sweetened this type of fish is a very valuable source of healthy fish oils.

Tip:

Fish cooks very quickly so try not to overcook it. Steamed, poached, baked or lightly sautéed is a much better option than fried or grilled. If you are worried about the mercury in the fish, eating three or four Brazil nuts with the fish will top up your supply of selenium.

Simple Baked Salmon with Two Sauces

SOME COOKED SALMON OR TROUT IN THE FREEZER IS A USEFUL STORE CUPBOARD INGREDIENT, SO IT IS WORTHWHILE COOKING A WHOLE SALMON OR A LARGE TROUT AND FREEZING IT, EITHER IN PORTIONS OR AS LARGE FLAKES. THESE DAYS, AS MOST OF US DO NOT OWN A FISH KETTLE, THE EASIEST WAY TO COOK A WHOLE SALMON IS IN THE OVEN, WRAPPED IN FOIL,. ALL YOU NEED TO DO BEFORE COOKING THE FISH IS TO HAVE THE SALMON CLEANED AND ITS SCALES REMOVED.

1 whole salmon weighing about
1.8Kg or 4 lb
1 tbsp olive oil
1 small white onion very finely sliced
3 – 4 fresh bay leaves
½ lemon finely sliced
A handful of parsley, chervil or dill
½ - 1 tsp crushed black pepper.

The slower the salmon is cooked the better the flavour. Pre heat the oven to 150°C/ 300°F/Gas 2

There is no need to wash the fish, just wipe it, inside and out, with some kitchen paper. Lay two large pieces of foil, one on top of the other and brush lightly with oil. Lay the fish on the foil and put the sliced onion, bay leaves, sliced lemon and herbs in the cavity. Fold the foil over the fish to make a loose parcel. Fold over the edges of the foil twice to seal it.

Place the parcel on a large baking sheet and bake the fish in the centre of the oven for 2½ hours. Remove it from the oven and leave it to cool in the foil.

The skin should come off easily when the fish is cooked and the fish should lift easily from the bones. If you are going to freeze some of the fish, portion it up and open freeze it in a single layer on a foil lined tray. Put it into into a box or bag after it is frozen.

Cooked Salad Dressing- Cheats Tartare Sauce

WITH MOST COMMERCIAL MAYONNAISE MADE FROM VEGETABLE OILS THAT ARE IN THE 'NEVER EAT' CATEGORY, THIS WAR TIME RECIPE FOR A COOKED SALAD DRESSING IS A USEFUL ALTERNATIVE. THE DRESSING WILL KEEP FOR 4 – 5 DAYS IN A JAR IN THE FRIDGE. YOU CAN USE IT JUST AS YOU WOULD COMMERCIAL MAYONNAISE AND BY ADDING SOME CHOPPED CAPERS, FINELY CHOPPED PICKLED GHERKINS AND SOME SNIPPED CHIVES YOU CAN QUICKLY TRANSFORM IT INTO A CHEATS TARTARE SAUCE.

1 tbsp plain flour OR cornflour
2 tsp mustard powder
1 tsp sugar
1 free range egg
1 tbsp olive oil or butter
175ml/6fl oz milk
4 tbsp lemon juice
A pinch of cayenne pepper
A pinch of garlic granules (optional)
FOR THE CHEATS TARTARE SAUCE
3 tbsp chopped capers
3 tbsp finely chopped pickled gherkins
1 tbsp finely chopped parsley or chervil
1 tbsp finely chopped chives

Mix together the flour, mustard powder, cayenne pepper and sugar. If you are using the adding the garlic granules add these also at this stage.

Beat the egg and milk together and whisk in the oil. If you are using butter melt it first. Slowly add this to the flour and mustard whisking everything until it is smooth.

Pour the mixture into a saucepan and bring it very slowly to the boil over a medium heat. Keep stirring all the time with the whisk to prevent it from sticking as it thickens.

Cook for 2 minutes. Leave it to cool and then whisk in the lemon juice. Season to taste with salt and pepper and extra lemon juice.

Caper & Coriander Vinaigrette

USE CORIANDER PESTO FROM THE FREEZER IF YOU DO NOT HAVE ANY FRESH CORIANDER

2 heaped tbsp finely chopped coriander
1 heaped tbsp capers roughly chopped
½ clove garlic crushed
1 spring onion finely sliced
1 tsp wholegrain mustard
2 tbsp olive oil
1 tbsp liquid from the capers
Salt and pepper to taste

Heat the oil in a small pan and lightly sauté the garlic and onion for 2 minutes. Add the rest of the ingredients and heat through.

Salmon Cured With Dill

GRAVLAX IS AN ANCIENT WAY OF CURING AND PRESERVING SALMON. MAKING YOUR OWN GRAVLAX IS SURPRISINGLY EASY. ONCE CURED THE SALMON KEEPS IN THE FRIDGE FOR UP TO A WEEK AND YOU CAN ALSO FREEZE IT FOR UP TO 3 MONTHS.

WHEN YOU LOOK AT THE RECIPE AND SEE THE AMOUNT OF SUGAR AND SALT THAT IT USES IT DOESN'T LOOK A HEALTHY OPTION, BUT THE SUGAR AND SALT ARE THERE ONLY TO EXTRACT THE FLUID FROM THE SALMON. ONCE THE CURING PROCESS HAS FINISHED VERY LITTLE IS LEFT IN THE FISH.

YOU WILL NEED A LARGE PIECE OF SALMON FROM THE MIDDLE OF THE FISH. THE SALMON NEEDS TO BE SCALED, FILLETED, BONED AND THEN PIN BONED. CLASSICALLY A GRAVLAX OF SALMON SHOULD WEIGHT ABOUT 1¼KG/2LB 13OZ.IF THE PIECE OF FISH YOU HAVE IS LARGER OR SMALLER JUST SCALE THE INGREDIENTS UP OR DOWN SO THAT THE RATIO OF SUGAR AND SALT TO FISH IS ABOUT THE SAME.

SERVES 6 - 8

1¼Kg/2lb 13oz fresh or previously frozen salmon
3 heaped tbsp dried dill
100g/3½oz sea salt crystals
85g/3oz sugar
2 tbsp crushed black or white peppercorns

You will need a container with a close fitting lid that is large enough to hold the salmon laid flat on its side.

If you are using frozen salmon leave it to thaw out over night. Wash it thoroughly and dry it with kitchen paper to remove any oil that may have gone rancid. If you are using fresh salmon, wipe it inside and out with damp kitchen paper and remove any blood from the inside.

Put the sugar, salt and crushed black pepper into a bowl and mix it together.

Put one side of the salmon into the container, spread the salt and sugar mixture over it and sprinkle on the dried dill. Put the other side of salmon on top. All you need to do now is put the lid on the container and then put the container into the fridge.

The salmon needs to be turned over twice a day and left to cure for 2 - 3 days depending on the thickness of the fish. As the salmon cures fluid will be drawn out of it. When you turn the salmon over baste the top and inside of the fish with this fluid. When the salmon has cured all you need to do is lift it from the cure and slice it thinly.

Cullen Skink

CULLEN SKINK IS A TRADITIONAL SCOTTISH FISH STEW WITH A HISTORY THAT GOES BACK HUNDREDS OF YEARS. YOU DO NOT NEED TO STICK RIGIDLY TO THE RECIPE AS YOU CAN MAKE THE SOUP FROM JUST ABOUT ANY FISH OR SHELLFISH THAT YOU HAVE AVAILABLE. HOWEVER, THE ONE THING YOU DO NEED TO INCLUDE IS SOME SMOKED FISH, PREFERABLY FISH THAT HAS BEEN NATURALLY SMOKED AND NOT DYED.

SERVES 4

1 large leek
1 medium onion
1 stick of celery very finely sliced
2 tbsp butter
2 tbsp plain flour
600ml/20fl oz (1pt) milk
300ml/10 fl oz (½pt) water
2 large potatoes peeled and cut into small cubes
450g/1lb un-dyed smoked haddock with skin and bones removed
115g/4oz small courgette cut into small dice
225g/8oz white fish with skin and bones removed
225g/8oz salmon with skin and bones removed
16 frozen mussels, shells removed

Trim the leek and discard any dark green leaves. Slice the leek and onion thinly.

Cut the fish into small 1cm/½in dice.

Melt the butter in a large saucepan and fry the leek, onion and celery over a medium heat for about 5 minutes.

Still with the pan on a medium heat, stir in the flour and cook it for 2 minutes stirring it occasionally, Be careful not to let it brown. Add the milk and water and stir until the liquid comes to the boil and thickens. If you have the heat too high the sauce at the bottom of the saucepan will stick and burn.

Add the potatoes and bring the soup slowly back to the boil. Reduce the heat to very low and simmer for 15 minutes or until the potatoes are tender.

Increase the heat a little and add the courgettes, the fish and the mussels and bring the soup to the boil. Turn the heat back to low and simmer for 5 – 7 minutes.

Season with black pepper and garnish with some finely chopped chives or chopped dill before serving.

Leek, Saffron & Mussel Soup

THIS RECIPE USES FROZEN MUSSELS AS THEY TAKE LESS TIME TO PREPARE AND ARE WIDELY AVAILABLE IN SUPERMARKETS. YOU CAN ALSO USE FRESH MUSSELS IN THEIR SHELLS IF YOU CAN GET THEM. IF YOU DO USE FRESH MUSSELS YOU WILL NEED ABOUT 1.5KG/3LB.

SERVES 4

300g/11oz frozen mussel meat, thawed, washed and dried

450g/16oz leeks coarsely chopped

5cm/2in piece white part of a leek cut into match stick size pieces

50ml/2 fl oz white wine OR Dry Vermouth (optional)

1 small onion chopped

50g/2oz butter

1tbsp flour

450ml/15 fl oz fish stock OR

450ml/15fl oz vegetable stock and 1Tbsp Thai fish sauce

A large pinch of saffron

50ml/2 fl oz fromage frais or natural unsweetened Greek yoghurt

Melt the butter in a saucepan and sauté the leeks and onion on a medium heat for 3 - 4 minutes. Be careful not to let them brown.

Stir in the flour and cook for 2 minutes. Add the stock and the saffron. If using vegetable stock and Thai fish sauce add the fish sauce just before you serve the soup. Bring everything to the boil, turn down the heat and simmer for 25 - 30 minutes.

Use a hand blender to purée the leeks and onion. At this stage you can turn off the heat or leave the soup simmering on a low heat.

When you are ready to serve the soup add the mussels, bring the soup to the boil and simmer gently for 5 minutes. Don't overcook the mussels as they will become tough.

Just before serving stir in the cream or yoghurt. Ladle the soup into individual bowls and garnish with the slices of leek.

Red Peppers Stuffed with Mackerel

MANY VEGETABLES LEND THEMSELVES TO BEING STUFFED AND THE INGREDIENTS YOU USE FOR THE STUFFING CAN BE QUITE VERSATILE. THIS RECIPE HAS ITS ORIGINS IN SPAIN WHERE COOKED SALT COD IS MIXED WITH MASHED POTATO AND USED TO STUFF ROASTED RED PEPPERS. TRADITIONALLY THE PEPPERS ARE SERVED WITH A SHELLFISH BISQUE. THIS A SIMPLE RECIPE THAT CAN BE PREPARED VERY QUICKLY. YOU CAN USE ANY TYPE OF FRESH OR CANNED FISH. THE FISH USED IN THIS RECIPE IS A 'NO DRAIN' CAN OF MACKEREL FILLETS THAT HAVE NO ADDED OIL. THIS TYPE OF FISH IS A USEFUL STORE CUPBOARD INGREDIENT.

SERVES 2

2 large red bell peppers
1 large potato weighing about 350g/12oz
110g/4oz tin 'no drain' mackerel fillets
1tsp chilli paste or Sambol Oelek
1 heaped tsp dried dill
2 - 3 spring onions finely sliced
50g/1¾oz prawns (optional)
1 tbsp Thai fish sauce

Pre heat the oven to 180°C/ 350°F/Gas 4

Prick the potato and cook it in a microwave on full power for 5 minutes. Turn it over and cook for another 3 -4 minutes until it is just soft.

As soon as the potato is cool enough to handle peel off the skin and either mash it or put it through a potato ricer.

Cut the peppers in half lengthways through the stem. Remove the seeds and any white pith.

Put the peppers cut side up into a lightly greased oven proof pan. You may need to trim the round side a little so that they sit flat. If you end up with a hole put the piece you trimmed off back inside to fill the gap.

Break the mackerel fillets into smallish chunks and mix them with the prawns, dill, spring onions, Sambol Oelek and Thai fish sauce into the mashed potato. Divide the mixture between the halved peppers and press it down well. Bake the peppers uncovered for 20 - 25 minutes or until they feel soft when tested with a sharp knife.

Fish Baked with Onion & Lemon

YOU CAN PREPARE THE ONION AND LEMON USED IN THIS DISH IN ADVANCE AND STORE IT IN THE FRIDGE FOR A DAY OR TWO. IT ALSO FREEZES WELL SO IT IS WORTH MAKING MORE THAN YOU NEED AND PUTTING SOME IN THE FREEZER FOR EMERGENCY USE. YOU CAN SERVE THE BAKED FISH WITH ANY TYPE OF GREEN VEGETABLE.

SERVES 4

350g/12oz white onion very finely sliced
4 cloves of garlic finely chopped
50g/1¾oz unsalted butter or ghee
75ml/2½ fl oz dry white wine.
Finely grated zest of a lemon
Juice of a lemon
Parsley, chervil or dill to garnish.
3 bay leaves
150ml/5 fl oz (¼ pt) fish stock
4 fillets of white fish weighing about 150g/5½oz each, skin and bones removed
400g/14oz butter beans drained and rinsed

You will need a large flame proof casserole or baking dish to cook this as the fish needs to be cooked in a single layer. If you do not have any fish stock use vegetable stock and a tablespoon of Thai fish sauce.

Use a potato peeler to thinly peel 3 pieces of rind from the lemon. Cut this into fine, paper thin slices. Grate the rest of the lemon rind.

Melt the butter in a saucepan and add the onion, garlic, bay leaves and grated lemon rind. Sauté over a medium heat for 5 minutes, then add the white wine. Cover and leave to cook very slowly over a low heat for 40 minutes. Stir it occasionally to prevent the onions sticking.

Pre heat the oven to 220°C/ 450°F/Gas 6.

Wash and dry the fish.

Remove the bay leaves and add the butter beans and the fish stock to the onions. Bring them to the boil and turn off the heat.

Pour the onion and stock into the casserole, place the pieces of fish on top and sprinkle on the thin slices of lemon zest. Cover with a lid or foil and bake for 20 minutes.

To serve, put a piece of fish on each plate, stir the lemon juice into the onion and butter beans and put a spoonful onto the plate. Garnish with chopped dill, parsley or chervil.

Classic Fish in Oatmeal with Beetroot Pesto

IF YOU ARE LUCKY ENOUGH TO BE ABLE TO BUY FRESH OILY FISH THIS IS A QUICK AND EASY WAY TO COOK IT. YOU CAN USE HERRING, SARDINES, MACKEREL OR TROUT. IF YOU ARE USING HERRING, MACKEREL OR TROUT YOU WILL NEED FISH THAT WEIGH ABOUT 300G/10½ OZ EACH WHEN WHOLE. IF YOU ARE USING SARDINES YOU WILL NEED 2 PER PERSON. YOU WILL FIND THE RECIPE FOR TOASTED OATMEAL COATING IN THE WHOLE GRAINS, SEEDS AND CEREALS SECTION.

NOTE: If you are using herrings or sardines ask the fishmonger to scale the fish as well as clean them. The fishmonger may also bone them for you but if you have to bone the fish yourself this is what you do.

Using a really sharp knife cut along the belly of the fish right down to the tail. Put the fish flesh side down onto a chopping board and use your hand to push down firmly to flatten it out. Then press very firmly along the back bone. This will loosen the backbone and the small bones that are attached to it. Turn the fish over, skin side down, and gently ease the back bone away. Most of the small fine bones will come away with it. Cut the back bone off just above the tail and trim around the belly to tidy the fish up. Use a piece of kitchen paper to wipe off any blood from the fish.

SERVES 2

2 herring, mackerel or trout or 4 sardines
About 85g/3 oz toasted oatmeal coating
2 tbsp flour for dusting
1 large free range egg
1 tbsp finely chopped capers
70g/2½ oz beetroot pesto
1 clove garlic (optional)

Pre heat the oven to 200°C/ 400°F/Gas 5

Put the toasted oatmeal coating into a blender and give it a quick whiz to break it down into smaller pieces. Break the egg into a wide shallow bowl and beat it.

You will need a baking tray that is large enough to lay the fish in a single layer. If the tray is non stick lightly bush it with oil otherwise line the tray with oiled baking foil. When the oven is hot put the tray in to get warm.

Dust both sides of the fish with seasoned flour, then dip the flesh side only in the beaten egg and then the oatmeal coating, pressing it down firmly. Lightly brush with some olive oil. Put to one side while you process the other fish.

Take the baking tray out of the oven and put the fish onto it oatmeal side down. Bake for 10 minutes. Take them out of the oven, turn them over and bake for another 5 minutes.

Beetroot Pesto

BEETROOT PESTO MAKES A COLOURFUL, TASTY DIP FOR VEGETABLES AND IT GOES REALLY WELL WITH SALMON, TROUT AND HERRING. YOU CAN ALSO STIR IT INTO QUINOA, BULGAR WHEAT AND PASTA. AS IT FREEZES WELL IT IS WORTH MAKING A BATCH FOR THE FREEZER.

250g/9oz packet of cooked beetroot roughly chopped
55g/2oz raw cashew nuts
Finely grated zest and juice of a lime
70g/2½oz finely grated parmesan
2 tbsp chopped parsley
3 heaped tsp grated horseradish
3 tbsp olive oil
Salt to taste
1 tbsp chopped capers
Crushed garlic to taste

Grind the cashew nuts in a food processor.

Put the capers to one side and add all of the other ingredients and blitz until everything is well mixed into to a paste. Omit the garlic if you are making the pesto for the freezer.

Put the pesto into a serving bowl and add the chopped capers. Serve the pesto in a separate bowl.

Creole Tuna Salad

THIS TUNA SALAD IS FAR REMOVED FROM THE TYPICAL TUNA SALAD. IT IS ONE OF THOSE SALADS THAT YOU CAN MAKE FROM MORE OR LESS ANY INGREDIENTS THAT YOU HAVE AVAILABLE AND IT IS MOST DEFINITELY MORE SALAD THAN FISH. YOU NEED GOOD QUALITY 'NO DRAIN' TUNA STEAK.

SERVES 2 – 4
1 large carrot coarsely grated
1 red pepper finely chopped
½ small red onion finely chopped
1 small green under ripe mango
Finely chopped chilli to taste
50g/1¾oz finely shredded cabbage or Chinese leaf
120g/4¼ oz can 'no drain' tuna steak in spring water
Finely grated zest and juice of a lime
2 tbsp chopped coriander or what ever herbs you have available
2 tbsp lightly toasted pumpkin and sunflower seeds

Remove the stone from the mango, then peel the mango and cut it into 1cm/½ in chunks. Put it into a large bowl and stir in the lime zest, lime juice and chopped chilli.

Add the grated carrot, red pepper, chopped onion and shredded cabbage.

Break up the tuna and stir it in. Garnish with the chopped herbs and toasted seeds. Serve with green or red Tabasco or hot pepper sauce.

Niçoise Salad

A CLASSIC WAY OF SERVING FRESH, FROZEN OR TINNED TUNA AND TRANSFORMING IT INTO A SUBSTANTIAL MEAL. YOU CAN VARY BOTH THE AMOUNT AND TYPE OF VEGETABLES YOU USE DEPENDING ON WHAT YOU HAVE AVAILABLE. IF YOU ARE USING FROZEN TUNA DEFROST IT SLOWLY AT ROOM TEMPERATURE AND THEN WASH AND DRY IT IN KITCHEN PAPER. DON'T BE PUT OFF BY THE LONG LIST OF INGREDIENTS. THIS IS A VERY EASY RECIPE TO MAKE.

SERVES 4

350g/12oz cherry tomatoes cut in half
110g/4 oz rocket or baby salad leaves
½ telegraph cucumber
175g/6oz fine French beans
450g/1lb cooked small new potatoes OR
400g/14oz can cannellini beans drained and rinsed
8 spring onions sliced
3 - 4 large free range eggs that have been hard boiled
1 tbsp finely chopped flat leaf parsley
20 salted black olives with their stones removed
400g/14oz tin 'no drain' tuna steak OR 4 x small pieces of fresh or frozen tuna

FOR THE DRESSING

Cooking fluid from the tuna
½ clove garlic crushed
1 tbsp seeded mustard
2 tbsp finely grated parmesan
1 tbsp lemon juice
1 heaped tsp anchovy paste

Cut each tuna steak in half horizontally into thin pieces.. Put 1 tbsp olive oil, 2 tbsp lemon juice and 2 tbsp water into a saucepan. Bring it to a gentle simmer and then add the pieces of tuna. Bring it back to simmering point, cover and cook for 3 minutes. Turn the slices of tune over and cook them for another 2 minutes. Take if off the heat and leave the tuna to cool while you prepare the salad.

Put the French beans into a pan of boiling water. Bring them to the boil and cook them for 3 minutes. Drain them, refresh them in cold water, drain them again and put them to one side.

Cut the cucumber in half lengthways and remove the seeds. Cut each half of the cucumber into thin crescent shaped slices.

Peel the hard boiled eggs and cut them into quarters.

Slice the cooked new potatoes into thin slices.

Put the French beans, tomatoes, sliced cucumber, potatoes, olives and spring onions into a bowl and mix well.

To make the dressing, drain the cooking liquid from the tuna into a jar and mix it with the anchovy paste, crushed garlic, seeded mustard, parmesan and lemon juice. Give it a really good shake to combine the ingredients.

When you are ready to serve the salad mix the rocket or the salad leaves with the other ingredients and arrange it on a serving plate. Put the pieces of tuna on top with the hard boiled eggs around the edge. Serve the parsley and dressing in separate bowls.

Fish Baked in Tomato & Cardamom Sauce

THIS RECIPE ORIGINATES FROM THE MIDDLE EAST. IT IS A BASIC TOMATO SAUCE THAT CAN BE USED WITH ANY TYPE OF WHITE FISH OR SHELLFISH.

SERVES 4

400g/14oz can chopped tomatoes
3 tbsp tomato purée
1 medium white or red onion chopped
1 tbsp olive oil
3 cloves garlic crushed
1 chopped chilli or 1 tsp Sambol Oelek
4 tbsp chopped fresh dill OR
2 tsp dried dill
2 tsp ground cumin
1 tsp ground cardamom
Ground black pepper to taste
4x fillets Tilapia or other white fish weighing about 150g/5½oz each

Pre heat the oven to 180°C/ 350°F/Gas 4

Heat the olive oil in a saucepan or frying pan. Add the onion and garlic and sauté for 3 – 4 minutes. Add the chilli or Sambol Oelek, the cardamom, the cumin and the dill, give it a good stir and then add the tinned tomatoes and the tomato purée. Leave the sauce to cook gently over a low heat while you prepare the fish.

Wash and dry the fish and put it into a greased baking dish that is large enough to lay the fish in a single layer.

Pour over the tomato sauce. Cover with foil and bake in the middle of the oven for 20 - 25 minutes depending on the thickness of the fish.

Tilapia Baked with Ginger, Soy & Sesame

SERVES 4

4 fillets of Tilapia or other white fish each weighing about 150g/5½oz
2 tbsp grated ginger
1 tbsp soy sauce
1 heaped tbsp toasted sesame seeds
3 cloves garlic crushed
2 spring onions chopped
2 tsp sesame oil
1 tbsp olive oil
Juice of a lemon

Pre heat the oven to 200°C/ 400°F/Gas 5

Heat the oil in a small saucepan, add the garlic, ginger and spring onions and sauté over a medium heat for 2 – 3 minutes. Be careful not to let them brown. Turn off the heat and mix in the soy sauce, sesame seeds, sesame oil and lemon juice. Put a quarter of the mixture into a small dish.

Wash and dry the fish and cut the fillets in half lengthways. If you are using tilapia you will have one thick piece and one thin piece.

Put a large piece of foil onto a baking sheet and lightly brush it with oil. Put the thick pieces of fish onto the foil, divide the sesame and ginger mixture between them and spread it out over the fillet. Put the thin pieces of fish on top and divide the rest of the sesame and ginger mixture between them. Cover with foil, put it into the middle of the oven and bake for 25 minutes.

Nuts & Seeds

Why?

All nuts and seeds contain different amounts of saturated, monounsaturated and polyunsaturated fats as well as protein, trace elements and fibre. They bring with them their own supply of antioxidants and vitamins that prevent the oils from oxidising. They are complex foods that contain many different phytonutrients, some of which are known to reduce chronic and systemic inflammation. Walnuts, almonds, hazelnuts, Brazil nuts, pumpkin seeds, sesame seeds, flax seeds, hemp seeds and chia seeds, in fact all nuts and seeds are good and they are great for snacking on.

All nuts and seeds contain Omega 3 and Omega 6 polyunsaturated fatty acids that are in a 'natural' ratio. Isn't Omega 6 one of the not so good fats? Well nuts and seeds are not just tiny packets of Omega 6. They are a long way from the heat processed polyunsaturated vegetable oils. However, when it comes to the Omega 3 fats things are not quite so straightforward. The 'parent' of the Omega 3 fats our body needs is ALA, alpha linoleic acid. This needs to be converted into EPA, eicosapentaenoic acid, and DHA, decosahexaenoic acid, before our bodies can use it. As this conversion process is extremely poor as little as 1% of the ALA we consume ends up as EPA or DHA. Unlike oily fish which contains large amounts of EPA and DHA in a readily available form, vegetable sources of Omega 3 fats only contain ALA, so after conversion we actually obtain only a very small amount of EPA and DHA from them. This is interesting as nuts and seeds, and chia seeds in particular, are being widely promoted as 'super foods' that are high in Omega 3. Sadly, this is in the form of ALA which is not a fat we can easily metabolise.

Notwithstanding this, as nuts and seeds are something a tree or plant grows from they are a pretty complete source of nutrition as they contain fats, carbohydrates and protein plus vitamins, minerals and antioxidants. When the oil is stripped from the nuts and seeds it doesn't have any of the antioxidants to protect it and this is when the trouble starts. A hand full of nuts or seeds is a very healthy food that bares no resemblance to a spoonful of hot pressed vegetable oil.

How?

Some people find raw nuts and seeds difficult to digest. Like all plants, grains, pulses and cereals, nuts and seeds contain anti-nutrients in one form or another. Phytic acid is the one most commonly found. Like all anti-nutrients this can inhibit the way in which we absorb minerals and trace elements and this can potentially lead to mineral deficiencies. Because of this there is something of a debate about whether you should remove these anti-nutrients before you eat the nuts and seeds.

Should you worry about anti nutrients like phytic acid? This really depends on how many nuts and seeds you consume and also when you eat them. If they are part of a meal the phytic acid will reduce the amount of minerals and trace elements you are able to absorb from it. However, if the nuts and seeds are eaten as a snack between meals the phytic acid will have little overall effect. So if you only eat a handful of nuts a day as part of an omnivorous diet it is unlikely to be a big deal. However, if you are a vegetarian or vegan eating nuts and seeds as a protein combined with pulses, lentils and whole grains then reducing your consumption of phytic acid could well be a good idea. There are three ways you can do this.

Roasting and cooking reduces the amount of phytic acid a food contains so roasting nuts and seeds or cooking them as part of a meal will reduce the amount of phytic acid you are consuming. It will also make the nuts and seeds easier to digest. However, only buy natural uncooked nuts and seeds. Commercially roasted nuts and seeds usually contain additives and you have no control over the temperature or the length of time they have been roasted for. Unless the packet specifically says 'dry roasted' as opposed to 'roasted', it is highly likely that the nuts will have been fried in polyunsaturated vegetable oil.

Another way of reducing the phytic acid content is to soak the nuts and seeds overnight. When you do this enzymes in the nuts and seeds begin to break down and remove the phytic acid and this is drained away with the soaking liquid. The nuts and seeds become plump and succulent and have more of a bite than a crunch.

Last but not least, is to eat the nuts and seeds with a lemon juice or vinegar dressing as lemon juice and vinegar increase the absorption of minerals and trace elements and this counters the effect of the phytic acid.

Celery & Almond Roast

THE UBIQUITOUS VEGETARIAN NUT ROAST BUT THIS IS A NUT ROAST WITH A DIFFERENCE. YOU CAN SERVE IT WITH TFAYA BUT IT ALSO WORKS WELL AS PART OF A MORE CONVENTIONAL 'ROAST DINNER'. YOU CAN USE SILKEN TOFU OR A LOW FAT CHEESE LIKE QUARK OR RICOTTA. THE ROAST CAN BE EATEN HOT OR COLD. IT DOES NOT FREEZE BUT IT WILL KEEP IN THE FRIDGE FOR 2 TO 3 DAYS.

SERVES 4 – 6

350g/12oz silken tofu
500g/1lb 2oz celery finely sliced
100g/3½oz flaked oats
4 tbsp finely grated parmesan
200g/7oz toasted flaked almonds
2 tbsp chopped parsley
½tsp ground turmeric
3 free range eggs
finely grated zest of a lemon
juice of a lemon

Heat the oven to 180°C/ 350°F/Gas 4

Put the finely sliced celery into a microwave bowl, cover and cook on full power for 5 minutes. Give it a stir, put the cover back on and cook for another 5 minutes. Leave it to cool slightly.

Put the flaked almonds onto a baking tray and bake them for 6 minutes. Just long enough for them to take on some colour.

Put the silken tofu into a large bowl, add the eggs, turmeric and lemon zest and give everything a whiz with a hand blender until the tofu is thoroughly amalgamated with the eggs.

Stir in the grated parmesan, the flaked oats, parsley, celery, toasted almonds and lemon juice.

Grease a 1½Kg/3lb 6oz loaf tin, spoon in the mixture and press it down. Cover with foil and bake for 30 minutes at 180°C/ 350°F/Gas 4.

Turn the oven down to 160°C/ 325°F/Gas 3, take off the foil and cook for another 30 minutes. Leave the roast to stand for 10 – 15 minutes before turning it out of the tin.

Brazil Nut & Vegetable Korma

A CREAMY LIGHTLY SPICED CURRY. LIKE MOST SPICED DISHES IT BENEFITS FROM BEING MADE IN ADVANCE SO THAT THE FLAVOURS CAN DEVELOP.

SERVES 4

50g/1¾oz creamed coconut
2 tbsp olive oil
2 medium onions chopped
2 fresh red or green chillies or2 tsp chilli paste
1 tsp ground cumin
1 tsp ground turmeric
1 tsp ground coriander
1 clove crushed garlic
125g/4 oz ground Brazil nuts or cashew nuts
1 small cauliflower broken into florets
250g/8 oz courgettes sliced
125g/4 oz sugar snaps
125g/4 oz cooked peas
4 tbsp fresh chopped coriander

Roughly chop the coconut and dissolve it in 450ml/16fl oz of boiling water. Heat the olive oil and fry the onion for 5 minutes, stirring occasionally. Add the chillies, garlic and spices. Stir well and cook for 2 minutes over a medium heat.

Stir the ground nuts into the coconut water and then add this to the onion and spices. Bring it to simmering point, cover and turn the heat to low. You can prepare the recipe to this stage and store it overnight in the fridge.

Put some water into a saucepan and bring it to the boil. Add the cauliflower and cook for 3 minutes. Stir in the sugar snaps, bring back to the boil, cover and turn off the heat.

While the cauliflower is cooking steam the courgettes in a microwave for 3 minutes.

Drain the cauliflower and sugar snaps and add them with the courgettes and cooked peas to the nut, spice and onion mixture. Serve garnished with chopped coriander.

Gomasio

Gomasio or Gomashio is a seasoning blend that is very nutritious. It tastes good sprinkled on stir fries, cooked vegetables and salads. It is very simple to make as the only ingredients are sesame seeds and a small amount of salt. You can use white, black or brown sesame seeds. For 15 table spoons of sesame seeds you will need 1 teaspoon of coarse sea salt crystals.

Heat a saucepan over a medium heat. Add the sesame seeds and toast them for just long enough to colour them slightly. You need to be patient and you need to keep stirring them to prevent them burning. Turn the heat down if they begin to take on colour quickly. How long toasting them will take depends on your saucepan and the type of seeds you are using. When they are ready they will start to pop and smell 'nutty'.

Leave the seeds to cool and when they are cold put them into a blender and grind them until about half of the seeds have been crushed. Add the sea salt crystals and give them a quick whiz to mix everything together and break down the salt crystals. As the Gomasio oxidises and becomes rancid very quickly after it is made, store it in an airtight container in the fridge.

Baked Aubergine with a Walnut Salsa

THIS IS AN UNUSUAL WAY OF SERVING AUBERGINE. AN ESSENTIAL INGREDIENT IS WALNUTS THAT HAVE BEEN PICKED BEFORE THE SHELLS HAVE FORMED AND THEN PICKLED. THEY GIVE THE SALSA ITS CHARACTERISTIC FLAVOUR. YOU CAN BUY THEM IN MOST LARGE FOOD STORES. THE AUBERGINES CAN BE EATEN HOT OR AT ROOM TEMPERATURE.

SERVES 4
2 large aubergines
2 tbsp olive oil
For the Salsa
85g/ 3oz chopped walnuts or pecan nuts
60g /2½oz pickled walnuts chopped into small pieces
85g/ 3oz crumbled feta or goats cheese
1 tbsp pickling liquid from the pickled walnuts
2 tbsp cider vinegar
1 clove garlic crushed
1 tsp Sambol Oelek or finely chopped red chilli
2 tsp walnut oil
1 tbsp chopped parsley
2 tbsp chopped coriander
1 tbsp pomegranate seeds OR 1 tsp of ground dried pomegranate seeds (optional)
100g/3½oz cooked quinoa (optional)

Pre heat the oven to 200°C/ 400°F/Gas 5.

Cut the aubergines in half lengthways. Put them onto a baking tray flesh side up and score the flesh in a criss-cross pattern. Brush them with oil, loosely cover with foil and bake for about 30 minutes until the flesh is soft and cooked through. Remove the aubergines from the oven and take off the foil.

To make the salsa, mix together the walnuts, the chopped pickled walnuts, the vinegar, oil, pickled walnut liquid, garlic, Sambol Oelek, the chopped parsley and half of the coriander. If you are using it stir in the cooked quinoa.

Spoon the salsa over the aubergine flesh. Just before serving add the crumbled feta and the remaining coriander. Lightly sprinkle with the powdered pomegranate seeds.

Goats Cheese & Walnut Salad

A SIMPLE CLASSIC SALAD THAT TAKES ONLY MINUTES TO PREPARE. IF YOU DON'T LIKE GOATS CHEESE USE CAMEMBERT OR BRIE INSTEAD.

SERVES 4

250g/9oz Chevre goats log cut into16 slices

16 thin slices from a small baguette

70g/2½oz mixed baby salad leaves

400g/14 oz can red beans drained and rinsed

85g/3oz walnuts or pecan nuts chopped

Small bunch chives finely chopped

FOR THE DRESSING

1 tbsp walnut oil

1 tbsp lemon juice

½ tsp chilli paste or Sambol Oelek

Set the grill onto high and toast the slices of baguette on one side.

Put the salad leaves into a large bowl with the red beans and the walnuts. Mix the walnut oil, chilli and lemon juice together and mix it into the salad and beans. Divide the salad between 4 plates.

Put the slices of Chevre onto the un-toasted side of the baguette and grill it until it turns a light golden brown. Keep an eye on it as it burns very easily.

Arrange 4 pieces of the grilled Chevre log on top of the salad and serve immediately.

Red Cabbage, Red Bean & Walnut Salad

THIS IS A VARIATION ON A TRADITIONAL RED BEAN AND WALNUT SALAD FROM THE CAUCUSES. WHILE IN NO WAY AUTHENTIC, THE PICKLED WALNUTS GIVE THE SALAD ITS CHARACTERISTIC FLAVOUR. IF YOU ARE UNABLE TO OBTAIN PICKLED WALNUTS INCREASE THE AMOUNT OF WALNUTS AND USE SOME WORCESTERSHIRE SAUCE INSTEAD OF THE PICKLED WALNUT VINEGAR.

SERVES 4

½ small red cabbage very finely shredded

1 medium red onion finely sliced

400g/14oz can red beans drained and rinsed

50g/1¾oz finely chopped walnuts

1 pickled walnut finely chopped

2 tbsp walnut oil

2 tbsp pickled walnut vinegar

1 tsp chilli paste or Sambol Oelek

1 clove garlic crushed (optional)

Juice and finely grated zest of a lime

2 tbsp finely chopped coriander OR 1 tbsp ready made coriander pesto

Mix together the walnuts, pickled walnuts, vinegar, walnut oil, chilli, lime juice, grated lime zest, crushed garlic and coriander.

Mix together the cabbage, red onion and beans, stir in the dressing, cover and chill.

The salad will keep for 2 days in a covered container in the fridge.

Hazelnut & Chocolate Spread

A HEALTHIER HOME MADE VERSION OF HAZELNUT AND CHOCOLATE SPREAD AND MAKING IT IS EASIER THAN YOU THINK.

200g/7oz hazelnuts
3 tbsp cocoa powder
3 heaped tbsp dark unrefined muscavado sugar
50g/1¾oz butter
1 tsp vanilla extract
2 tbsp water + 6 tbsp water

Pre heat the oven to 180°C/ 350°F/Gas 4

Put the hazelnuts onto a baking tray and roast them for precisely 8 minutes. This will bring out their flavour.

Take them out of the oven, put them into a damp tea towel and rub them. Most of the skins will come off, don't worry about any that are left on.

Put the nuts into a food processor or blender and pulse them until you have a fine powder. The powder will work its way up the sides of the food processor so every now and then take off the lid and scrape them back down.

Keep processing. The nuts will begin to form a stiff lumpy mass. Carry on processing until the nuts begin to release their oil and form a smooth paste. This will take between 5 and 10 minutes or slightly longer and the paste will become slightly warm. Now prepare the chocolate.

Put 2 tbsp water, the butter, the cocoa powder and the sugar into a small saucepan and gently heat it until the butter is melted. Keep stirring it over a low heat and cook it for 3 – 4 minutes. This will take the raw taste out of the cocoa.

Stir in 1 tsp vanilla extract and leave the mixture to cool slightly.

Pour the chocolate mixture into the hazelnuts and process. Slowly add 6 tbsp cold water, 1 tbsp at a time until you have a smooth slightly runny paste.

You can keep the hazelnut and chocolate spread in a covered container in the fridge for several days or you can freeze it in portion size amounts.

Onion & Walnut Muffins

THESE SAVOURY MUFFINS ARE GREAT FOR BREAKFAST AND THEY ALSO GO REALLY WELL WITH SOUP. IF YOU ARE AVOIDING WHEAT USE A MIXTURE OF FINE OATMEAL AND BUCKWHEAT FLOUR INSTEAD OF THE SPELT. THESE MUFFINS FREEZE WELL

Makes 8 large muffins or 12 small ones
125g/4½oz white onion roughly chopped
4 tbsp olive oil
1 large free range egg
1 tsp cayenne pepper
1 tsp garlic granules
1 tsp baking powder
150g/5½oz finely chopped pecan nuts or walnuts
175g/6oz wholegrain spelt

Pre heat the oven to 220°C/ 450°F/Gas 6 and grease your muffin tins.

Put the walnuts into a blender or food processor and process until they are finely chopped. Put them into a bowl with the spelt and baking powder and mix well.

Put the chopped onion with the olive oil, egg, cayenne pepper and garlic granules into a food processor or blender and whiz until you have a smooth purée.

Add the onion and egg purée to the walnut and spelt and mix thoroughly. Spoon into the muffin tins and bake for 5 minutes then turn the oven down to 200°C/ 400°F/Gas 5 and cook for another 15 minutes.

White, Green and Oolong Tea

White, green and oolong tea has been around for a very long time and it has been the staple drink of millions of people in China and Japan for thousands of years. Today these teas are the world's most widely consumed beverage after water. While the Chinese and Japanese have known about its health giving properties for years, it is only recently that science has discovered why this type of tea is such a good thing to drink.

Why?

White, green and oolong teas really are healthy drinks and they need to be included in a healthy diet. These types of tea contain B vitamins, folic acid, manganese, potassium and magnesium and they are loaded with antioxidants in the form of flavonoids and polyphenols. Five of the flavonoids in green tea are called catechins and these are highly potent antioxidants. One of these, Epigallocatechin Gallette is thought to be twice as powerful as Resveratrol, the polyphenol that is found in red grapes. Some research has shown that this type of tea has greater antioxidant capability than Vitamin C and Vitamin E. Green, white and oolong teas also help regulate blood sugar and there is strong evidence that because of the powerful antioxidants they contain, as well as reducing total cholesterol levels, they also improve the ratio of HDL to LDL cholesterol.

What exactly is tea?

All types of tea, irrespective of whether they are green, white, oolong or black, start out as the green leaves of a plant called Camellia Sinensis. The only difference between them is the type of leaves that are used, where the tea is grown, when the leaves are picked and how the leaves are fermented, processed and dried. Unlike black tea all green, white and oolong teas are 'brewed' before being drunk without milk or sugar. As Asian people consume very few dairy products these teas have traditionally always been drunk this way, but it is thought that the casein in milk can bind to one of the most powerful catechins in the tea and reduce its antioxidant effect.

All green, white and oolong teas are made with water that is below boiling point. The low temperature means that the antioxidant and anti-inflammatory compounds the teas contain are not damaged during the brewing process. The tea is always made very weak and drunk very fresh, when it has a bright and vibrant colour. As the tea stands its colour darkens as it begins to oxidise. Different types of tea contain different amounts of catechins; green and white teas contain between 15% and 30%, oolong between 8% and 20% and black tea between 3% and 10%. You can drink as much of this type of tea as you want and it is an excellent way of keeping yourself well hydrated.

Matcha

Over the last year or two drinking green tea in the form of Matcha, has become one of the fastest growing health trends. As a result it is now a big talking point on health and wellness web sites. Matcha, which is traditionally made from the Japanese tea Sencha, is different to conventional green tea as the tea plants that are used to make it are shaded from the sun for three weeks before the leaves are harvested. The stems and veins are also removed before the leaves are processed. During the period of shaded growth the tea bush produces more theanine and caffeine. These two compounds are known to have the ability to increase natural levels of serotonin, dopamine, GABA and glycine, all of which are known to reduce mental stress. This accounts for the calming effect people say they experience when drinking Matcha.

When you are drinking Matcha, you are drinking ground powdered leaves that are suspended in water and this is very different to ordinary green tea where the leaves are steeped and then removed. As a result Matcha is highly concentrated and contains around three times more antioxidants than ordinary green tea. Because of world demand China is now producing a green tea that is being sold as Matcha. As this is not authentic there are inevitably questions about its quality so if you want to try Matcha make sure you buy Japanese Matcha made from Sencha tea.

How?

You will find green, white and oolong teas in most Chinese and Asian supermarkets. You can also buy them on the internet. The quality of tea varies enormously, as does its price. Just remember that a little goes a long way. Just a few grams are needed to make a large pot and you can obtain two and sometimes three 'brews' out of the same leaves. Because of its new found popularity you should be able to buy Matcha in most food stores and supermarkets but it is expensive, about £20 or $30 for 30g and 30g will only make around 20 cups of tea.

How you make green, white and oolong tea is critical. Different types of tea need to be made with water at different temperatures. If it is too hot the tea can taste bitter, even burnt and be unpleasant to drink. Making it with filtered or bottled water is a good idea as it this brings out the full flavour of the tea and gives it a lighter and brighter colour.

Green, White and Oolong teas have beautiful colours so drink them from a glass, not a cup or mug. Try adding some slices of lemon or ginger to the tea and then leaving it to cool. The lemon and ginger compliment the flavour and prevents the tea from oxidising, so the tea retains its colour.

Herbs and Spices

Why?

Herbs and spices have been around for thousands of years and they form a major part of the diet of many countries. Indian, Asian and North African food all gain their characteristic flavours from herbs and spices. When it comes to eating a healthy diet herbs and spies are close to being a secret weapon because as well as adding flavour to your food they are also packed full of phytonutrients. These have powerful antioxidant, anti-inflammatory and medicinal properties. Chilli peppers, rosemary, ginger, cinnamon, bay leaves, cumin, turmeric, coriander, dill, fennel, garlic, oregano, chervil, parsley, sage, thyme and tarragon are all great and their use in cooking as well as medicine goes back a long way. The active ingredient in turmeric called curcumin is a very strong antioxidant and an extremely powerful anti-inflammatory. Parsley and chervil have attracted a lot of attention recently as they are both very rich sources of flavonoids, Vitamin C, Vitamin K and the beta carotene which is needed to make Vitamin A as well as some very powerful oils. Interestingly, in the middle ages, parsley and chervil were used extensively by the monks in their herbal medicines.

How?

Herbs like basil, parsley, coriander, tarragon and herb rocket make really good pesto and this is an excellent way of concentrating their health giving properties. The classic Italian paste of gremolatta is basically parsley, lemon zest and garlic and it tastes delicious. When you use pesto you add a completely new dimension to your food. Pesto freezes really well in small pots. Just remember to add any garlic after you have thawed it out, not before, as when it is frozen garlic can develop off flavours that to some can taste unpleasant.

Tip:

Use fresh herbs whenever possible. Dried herbs just don't taste the same. Avoid cooking herbs, especially herbs like basil, dill, coriander, chervil and parsley. It changes their flavour as well as reducing their nutritional benefits so add them to your food at the last minute. Freezing herbs is the best way of preserving them as their nutritional value is not damaged and their flavour is only slightly changed.

Making Pesto

Making pesto is a little time consuming and it is certainly not something you want to do every day, so if you are going to make some it is worth making a large batch and freezing it in small portions. Just remember to leave out the garlic. You can always add garlic when you thaw the pesto out.

How do you freeze pesto? All you need to do is open freeze large spoon fulls on a tray lined with cling film and when the pesto is frozen store it a small bag or freezer box. If you make large amounts of pesto it is worthwhile investing in some small silicon muffin tins and using these to hold the pesto while it is being frozen.

Basil Pesto

THE 'PESTO' WE ALL THINK OF AS PESTO. LIKE CORIANDER PESTO, THIS IS SO USEFUL IT IS WORTH MAKING IT IN LARGE QUANTITIES. MOST RECIPES FOR BASIL PESTO USE PINE NUTS BUT ANY TYPE OF NUT WILL DO.

300g/10½oz basil
100g/3½oz raw cashew nuts
30g/1oz lightly toasted sunflower seeds
10 tbsp olive oil
85g/3oz finely grated parmesan
Crushed garlic to taste

Wash and dry the basil and remove any coarse stems. Put the cashew nuts and sunflower seeds into a food processor and grind them.

Add the basil to the food processor. You will need to do this in stages as there will be too much basil to go in in one go. When the basil has reduced in volume add the other ingredients and blend well.

Rocket Pesto

100g/3½oz rocket
50g/1¾oz grated parmesan
½ tsp grain mustard
1 tsp Sambol Oelek or chilli paste
Juice ½ lemon
1 tbsp white wine vinegar
50g/1¾oz ground almonds
4 tbsp olive oil
Crushed garlic to taste

Wash and dry the rocket and remove any tough leaves. Put everything into a food processor and blend until fully mixed.

Coriander Pesto

HAVING CORIANDER PESTO IN THE FREEZER IS REALLY USEFUL, ESPECIALLY WHEN YOU ARE MAKING AND SERVING CURRIES AND MEXICAN FOOD.

175g/6oz coriander leaves and stems
3 tbsp whole almonds with their skins
4 tbsp olive oil
Salt to taste
Finely grated zest oand juice of a lime
1 tsp finely chopped chilli OR 1 tsp Sambol Oelek

Wash and dry the coriander. Grind the almonds to a fine powder in a blender or food processor. Roughly chop the coriander and add it with the other ingredients to the almonds in the food processor and blend until fully mixed.

Gremolata

THIS IS AN ADAPTATION OF THE CLASSICAL ITALIAN GREMOLATA WHICH IS A MIXTURE OF VERY FINELY CHOPPED PARSLEY AND LEMON JUICE. YOU CAN USE ANY TYPE OF NUT BUT MAKE SURE YOU USE FLAT LEAF PARSLEY AND NOT CURLED PARSLEY AS IT HAS A MUCH BETTER FLAVOUR. MIXED WITH TOASTED OATMEAL COATING OR PANKO BREADCRUMBS IT MAKES A REALLY GOOD TOPPING FOR BAKES AND VEGETABLES.

250g/9 oz flat leaf parsley
50g/1¾oz walnuts or pecan nuts
3 tbsp olive oil
1 tbsp finely grated parmesan
Finely grated zest of a lemon
Juice of a lemon
Garlic and salt to taste

Remove any coarse stems from the parsley and then wash and drain it. If necessary dry it in some kitchen paper. Roughly chop it.

Grind the walnuts to a fairly fine powder in a food processor.

Add all the other ingredients and blend until everything is well mixed into a thick purée.

Pesto & Pickled Red Onion Salad

THIS IS ONE OF THOSE FLEXIBLE SALADS THAT CAN BE MADE WITH POTATOES, BUTTER BEANS OR CANNELLINI BEANS AND MORE OR LESS ANY SALAD VEGETABLES THAT YOU HAVE AVAILABLE. THE PICKLED RED ONIONS AND PESTO GIVE THIS SALAD A SPECIAL TWIST. THESE PICKLED RED ONIONS ARE A USEFUL ADDITION TO ALL TYPES OF SALADS AND BAKED VEGETABLE DISHES. THEY CAN BE MADE IN ADVANCE AND KEPT IN THE FRIDGE FOR SEVERAL DAYS.

SERVES 4 - 6

6 pickled baby red onions
12 small cooked salad potatoes
225g /8oz cooked French beans
6 small cooked artichoke hearts
6 spring onions shredded
30g/1oz basil pesto
Juice of half a lemon
3 tbsp fluid from the red onions
1 clove of crushed garlic (optional)
125g / 4oz baby plum tomatoes cut into halves
18 stoned black olives
80g/3oz baby salad leaves or rocket
parmesan flakes

FOR THE PICKLED RED ONIONS
450g / 1 lb small red onions
90ml / 3 fl oz olive oil
90ml / 3 fl oz balsamic vinegar
Juice of a lemon

First make the pickled red onions. Peel the onions. If they are small, about the size of a large walnut, leave them whole, otherwise cut them in half or quarters.

Bring a pan of water to the boil. Add the onions, bring the water back to the boil and simmer the onions for 2 minutes. Drain and add the balsamic vinegar and olive oil. Add the juice of one lemon and optionally some zest of the lemon peeled and cut into strips. Season with ground black pepper.

Leave the onions to marinade, turning every now and again. Leave them for at least 3 hours before serving.

To make the salad. Cut the potatoes into halves and squeeze the juice of half a lemon over them. Cook the French beans for 2 to 3 minutes until just al dente. Drain and refresh them in cold water.

To make the dressing, mix the pesto with the crushed garlic and the fluid from the pickled red onions.

Mix all the ingredients other than the salad leaves together and stir in the dressing. Add the salad leaves just before serving. Finish the salad with the parmesan flakes.

Carrots with Saffron & Cumin

CARROTS ARE NATURALLY QUITE SWEET AND BRAISING THEM BRINGS OUT THEIR NATURAL SWEETNESS. YOU CAN USE ANY TYPE OF CARROT BUT YOUNG NEW SEASON CARROTS ARE PARTICULARLY GOOD. YOU CAN SERVE THIS DISH ON ITS OWN, WITH FIRM TOFU OR WITH COOKED CHICKPEAS ADDED AT THE END. YOU CAN ALSO TURN IT INTO A DELICIOUS SOUP SIMPLY BY ADDING SOME MORE WATER AND BLENDING IT UNTIL IT IS SMOOTH.

SERVES 4

500g/1lb 2oz carrots peeled
3 tbsp olive oil
1 tsp ground cumin
1 tsp cumin seeds
Generous pinch of saffron
150ml/5 fl oz (¼ pt) water
1 tsp vegetable stock powder
4 large cloves of garlic finely sliced
Finely grated zest of half a lemon plus the
juice of half a lemon
Salt and ground black pepper
400g/14oz tin chick peas (optional)
2 tbsp chopped dill to garnish

Put the saffron to soak in 2 tbsp hot water while you prepare the carrots. Warm the water and dissolve the vegetable stock in it.

If the carrots are small leave them whole. If they are large either cut them into quarters lengthways or cut them across at a diagonal to form oval slices about ½cm/¼ in thick.

Heat the oil in a large saucepan and add the ground cumin, cumin seeds and sliced garlic. Stir briefly and then add the carrots, stirring constantly to coat them with the oil and spices.

Add the saffron and its soaking liquid, the stock and the lemon zest. Bring to the boil, turn down the heat, cover and simmer for about 15 - 20 minutes until the carrots are tender.

The precise cooking time will depend on the size and age of the carrots. New season carrots will cook more quickly. Stir the carrots every 5 minutes to make sure that they do not stick. When the carrots are tender you should have a fairly thick, slightly sticky sauce.

Add the tofu or the chickpeas if you are using them and heat through. Stir in the lemon juice just before serving and garnish with chopped dill.

Spicy Carrot Soup

YELLOW THAI CURRY IS MADE FROM CHILLIES, TURMERIC, GINGER AND GARLIC. YOU CAN BUY THAI CURRY PASTE ON LINE AND IN ASIAN SUPERMARKETS.

SERVES 4

1 large white onion finely sliced
1 tbsp olive oil
700g/1 lb 8 oz carrots
1Lt/35 fl oz vegetable stock
100g/3½oz red lentils
1 tbsp yellow Thai curry paste
3 handfuls of coriander finely chopped

Peel and slice the carrots into 5ml/¼in rounds.

Heat the olive oil over a medium heat and add the onion. Sauté for a minute or two. Add the Thai curry paste and the sliced carrots and stir for a minute or two.

Add the vegetable stock and the lentils. Turn up the heat and bring the soup to the boil, stirring occasionally to prevent the lentils sticking.

Turn the heat to low, cover and simmer for 30 minutes.

When you are ready to serve, blitz the soup with a hand blender and stir in half of the chopped coriander. Serve the rest of the coriander in a separate bowl.

Yogurt, Milk & Dairy Products

Why?

While many people thrive on dairy products others are unable to cope with them. If you are one of the people who thrives on them go ahead and enjoy them. They are a highly nutritious food that provides us with calcium, vitamins C, D, B1, B2 and B6 as well as potassium, phosphorous, selenium, zinc and magnesium. A 250ml cup of milk contains 146 kcal, 8 grams of fat, 8 grams of protein and 13 grams of carbohydrate. So calorie for calorie milk is highly nutritious. It contains a little bit of just about everything we need. However this comes with the caveat of how the cows that produce the milk are reared. Milk from grass fed cows is nutritionally very different to the milk from cows that are intensively reared and fed on grain.

Despite the dire warnings about saturated fat it is interesting to note that full fat dairy products, irrespective of whether they come from cows, sheep or goats, are associated with a lower risk of obesity and type 2 diabetes, improved insulin sensitivity and lower levels of triglycerides.

How?

You can drink milk and eat yoghurt at any time, but only eat yogurt that is natural, unflavoured, unsweetened, not thickened, not pasteurised and not fat reduced. It needs to be 'alive and kicking' with acidophilus, bifidus and other healthy bacteria.

Yoghurt makes a really good start to the day mixed with nuts and oatmeal. Add your own fruit, without sugar. Use yoghurt to make smoothies using whole fruit. You can use yoghurt for dressings instead of mayonnaise and flavoured with lime zest and herbs it makes a wonderful addition stirred into soup. Try mixing it with grated cucumber, carrot or mint and using it as a dip for vegetables.

Cottage cheese, curd cheese, hard cheese and cream are all good. By cheese I mean real cheese that has a texture, comes with rind and tastes of something, not the processed dyed stuff that comes in orange or yellow slabs. Camembert and blue cheeses like Roquefort and Stilton are all good. If you can obtain it try goat or sheep cheese. They both have a very pronounced flavour so you eat much less of them. Hard cheeses like parmesan and pecorino have intensely strong flavours and a little grated over your food goes a long way. Have a go at making your own ice cream but go easy on the sugar.

Pumpkin & Roquefort Torte

THIS RECIPE CAME FROM ONE OF THOSE 'WHAT HAVE I GOT IN THE FRIDGE' MOMENTS. YOU CAN USE PUMPKIN OR BUTTERNUT SQUASH, ANY TYPE OF BLUE CHEESE. YOU CAN EAT THE TORTE EITHER HOT OR COLD.

SERVES 6 – 8

350g/12oz Ricotta, Quark or other low fat cheese
3 large free range eggs
150g/5½oz Roquefort or other blue cheese
600g/1lb 5oz pumpkin or 1 medium butternut squash
225g/8oz cauliflower broken into small florets

You will need a 24cm/10 in silicon cake tin or spring form tin with a loose base to make this. If you are using an ordinary tin grease it well.

Pre heat the oven to 220°C/ 450°F/Gas 6

There is no need to peel the pumpkin, just cut it into wedges. If you are using butternut squash, again there is no need to peel it, just cut it in half length ways. Lightly oil a large pan or baking tray and put the pumpkin in a single layer or place the butternut squash cut side down. Bake the pumpkin for 20 minutes. The butternut squash will probably need 30 minutes. Take it out of the oven and leave it to cool.

Turn the oven down to 180°C/ 350°F/Gas 4

Put the cauliflower into a microwave bowl with a couple of tablespoons of water, cover and cook on full power for 5 minutes. Drain and put to one side.

When the pumpkin or butternut squash is cool enough to handled take off the skin and cut it into 2½cm / 1in chunks.

Mix the Ricotta or Quark, Roquefort cheese and the eggs together using a hand blender. Stir in the pumpkin (or butternut squash) and the cauliflower, pour it into the greased baking tin, put it in the oven and bake for 15 minutes.

Cucumber & Yoghurt Salad

THIS IS A VERY SIMPLE SALAD TYPE DIP THAT IS MADE FROM GRATED CUCUMBER AND YOGHURT. THIS BASIC COMBINATION OF INGREDIENTS IS FOUND ALL OVER THE WORLD. IN GREECE IT IS FLAVOURED WITH GARLIC AND DILL AND CALLED TZATZIKI AND IN INDIA IT IS FLAVOURED WITH MINT AND CALLED RAITA.

1 large telegraph cucumber or
300g/11oz Lebanese cucumbers
½ tsp salt
1 - 2 cloves crushed garlic
1 tsp dried dill or more to taste
300ml/10 fl oz thick natural unsweetened yoghurt

The secret of making this and any other type of cucumber salad is to remove as much water as possible from the cucumber. In order to do this you will need an clean tea towel or some muslin.

Place the tea towel or muslin on a deep plate and coarsely grate the cucumber onto it. Gather up the tea towel and squeeze out as much of the fluid from the cucumber as you can. You will be amazed how much comes out.

Put the cucumber into a bowl and add ½ teaspoon of salt, a clove of crushed garlic and the dried dill. Give it a good stir and then add about two thirds of the yoghurt. Stir it round and if the mixture looks too thick add the rest of the yoghurt. How much you need to add depends on how much fluid was in the cucumber in the first place and how much you have managed to squeeze out. Add more garlic to taste.

Chocolate & Raspberry Fromage Frais

THIS IS PROBABLY ONE OF THE QUICKEST AND EASIEST DESSERTS YOU CAN MAKE.

SERVES 4
120g/5 oz dark chocolate
150g/5 oz raspberries, fresh or frozen
2 tsp finely grated zest of a lemon
300g/10½oz fromage frais

Break the chocolate into pieces and put it into a small dry bowl. Put the bowl on top of a saucepan of gently simmering water and leave it to melt slowly.

Take the bowl off of the saucepan, stir in the lemon zest and leave the chocolate to cool for 15 minutes.

Stir the fromage frais into the chocolate and then gently stir in the raspberries. Spoon it into glasses. Chill well before serving.

Cranachan

A TRADITIONAL SCOTTISH DESSERT MADE FROM TOASTED OATMEAL. THE OATMEAL IS SOAKED OVERNIGHT IN WHISKEY AND HONEY AND THEN MIXED WITH SOFT CHEESE AND RASPBERRIES. MOST RECIPES YOU SEE TODAY DO NOT SOAK THE OATMEAL AND THEY USE WHIPPED CREAM INSTEAD OF THE CHEESE. THIS RECIPE USES HALF FROMAGE FRAIS AND HALF THICK GREEK YOGHURT INSTEAD OF THE CREAM BUT YOU COULD ALSO USE A SOFT LOW FAT CHEESE LIKE RICOTTA OR QUARK. THE WHISKEY GIVES THE DESSERT ITS CHARACTERISTIC FLAVOUR. WHETHER YOU USE WHISKEY AND HOW MUCH YOU USE IS A MATTER OF PERSONAL TASTE.

SERVES 4
300ml/10 fl oz (½pt) fromage frais
300ml/10 fl oz (½pt) thick unsweetened Greek yoghurt
85g/3 oz flaked oats that have been toasted golden brown
3 tbsp Whiskey
3 tbsp runny honey
450g/1lb raspberries
Toasted flaked almonds to garnish

Mix 2 tbsp of the honey and 2 tbsp of the whiskey with the toasted oatmeal and leave it to soak.. How long you soak it for is a matter of taste. The longer it soaks the softer it becomes.

Beat the fromage frais and yoghurt together until they are thoroughly blended and then stir in the remaining honey and whisky.

Crush half of the raspberries lightly with a fork and stir them into the yoghurt mixture.

Put a layer of whole raspberries into the bottom of 4 dessert glasses. Put in a layer of the yoghurt mixture and then a layer of the oatmeal. Continue until you have used all the raspberries. Finish with a layer of yoghurt.

Garnish with the toasted flaked almonds before serving.

Pumpkin, Tomato & Chestnut Bake with Tapenade

A SIMPLE DISH THAT LOOKS GREAT, TASTES GREAT AND IS QUICK AND EASY TO PREPARE. YOU CAN USE PUMPKIN, BUTTERNUT SQUASH OR SWEET POTATOES TO MAKE THIS. THE RECIPE FOR TAPENADE IS IN THE OLIVES AND OLIVE OIL SECTION.

SERVES 4

1½ Kg/3lb 6 oz pumpkin or butternut squash
1 tsp oregano
1 tsp chilli flakes
1 tbsp olive oil
200g/7oz cherry tomatoes
2 balls mozzarella cheese cut into slices OR a handful of finely shaved parmesan
Small handful of basil leaves
12 cooked chestnuts cut into quarters
2 tbsp balsamic vinegar
60g/2¼oz packet baby spinach or rocket leaves
Black olive Tapenade

Pre heat the oven to 200°C/ 400°F/Gas 5

Peel the pumpkin or butternut squash, remove the seeds and chop it into large chunks.

Put it into a bowl and add the olive oil, oregano and chilli flakes and season to taste.

Put the pumpkin or butter squash onto a roasting tray lined with non stick foil and bake for 15 minutes. Add the cherry tomatoes and the chestnuts and turn them over with the pumpkin or squash. Cook for another 10 minutes.

Stir in the basil leaves and the mozzarella or shaved parmesan and drizzle over the balsamic vinegar.

Serve on a bed of rocket or baby spinach with some black olive tapenade on the side.

Eggs

Why?

Eggs are an excellent source of protein, vitamins, trace elements and essential fatty acids. In fact when it comes to nutrients there is very little that eggs do not have and they are top of the list when it comes to bio availability. However, in order to ensure that you have a healthy ratio of Omega-3 to Omega-6 make sure you buy free range eggs from hens that spend their life running around in a field. The nutritional content of a free range egg, especially its Omega-3 content, is totally different to an egg from a hen that is kept in a battery farm. You do not need to buy Omega-3 enriched eggs either. All this means is that the poor battery hen has been fed on fish meal. The eggs from the happy hens will have just as much Omega-3.

Eggs are bad for me, they contain a large amount of cholesterol?

Yes its true, they do contain a large amount of cholesterol. A large boiled egg weighs around 50 grams and it contains around 200mg of cholesterol. The same 50 gram portion of lean beef contains around 40mg of cholesterol. It is the same old myth about saturated fats. Eggs contain many healthy things as well as cholesterol. When they form part of a balanced diet that is rich in vegetables, complex carbohydrates, antioxidants and fibre they are fine.

When it comes to eggs we have been well and truly brain washed. Eggs are so bad for us we eat sugary breakfast cereal instead of eggs for breakfast!! But eggs have been part of our diet for thousands of years. If you search the internet you will find plenty of sites expounding the dangers of eating eggs. Eat a maximum of two a week, up to one a day is 'safe'. The bottom line in the *"eggs are bad for you story"* is that they have been tainted by association with the bad company they keep on our plate. It is processed sausage, bacon, bread and hash brownies fried in vegetable oil that are the problem, not the eggs.

How?

Boil or poach them, scramble them lightly in butter or use them in an omelette. Just avoid frying them in polyunsaturated vegetable oil. Use butter, olive oil, lard or coconut oil instead. Mixed with vegetables like spinach, cauliflower, courgettes, peppers, pumpkin and butter nut squash they make great tortillas and frittatas.

Egg Soubise

SOUBISE IS A THICK CREAMY SAUCE THAT IS TRADITIONALLY MADE WITH ONIONS AND CREAM. THIS RECIPE IS QUICK AND EASY TO PREPARE. IT CAN BE SERVED WITH ANY TYPE OF VEGETABLE OR A SIMPLE SALAD. WITHOUT THE BOILED EGGS THE SOUBISE WILL KEEP IN THE FRIDGE FOR A COUPLE OF DAYS. IT CAN ALSO BE FROZEN. YOU CAN IF YOU WISH ADD SOME COOKED MUSSELS TO THE SOUBISE JUST BEFORE YOU PUT IT INTO THE OVEN. THIS WORKS PARTICULARLY WELL IF THE SOUBISE IS MADE FROM LEEKS INSTEAD OF ONIONS.

SERVES 4

750g/1lb 10oz white onions sliced
1 tbsp butter
3 tbsp milk
Finely grated zest and juice of ½ lemon
2 bay leaves
2 tbsp Japanese panko breadcrumbs
300ml/10 fl oz (½pt) fromage frais or Greek style natural unsweetened yoghurt
6 large free range eggs that have been hard boiled.
Crushed black pepper to taste

Heat the butter in a saucepan and gently sauté the onions over a medium heat for 5 minutes. Stir in the milk, the bay leaves and lemon zest, cover the saucepan, reduce the heat to low and simmer the onions for 30 minutes until they are soft. Leave them to cool slightly.

Pre heat the oven to 180°C/ 350°F/Gas 4

Peel the eggs and cut them in half. Put them cut side down either in individual dishes or in a single layer in a baking dish.

Remove the bay leaves and add the yoghurt, crushed black pepper and lemon juice to the onions. Purée them using a hand blender. Stir in the breadcrumbs and pour the purée over the eggs. Bake for 20 minutes.

Not Quite An Arnold Bennett Omelette

TRADITIONALLY AN ARNOLD BENNETT OMELETTE IS AN OMELETTE FOR 2 PEOPLE THAT IS TOPPED WITH SMOKED HADDOCK AND A CREAMY BÉCHAMEL SAUCE. THIS IS A MORE SUBSTANTIAL VERSION THAT USES SALMON OR TROUT AND COURGETTE TO TURN THE OMELETTE INTO A MEAL FOR 4 PEOPLE. YOU CAN USE ANY CUT OF SALMON OR TROUT TO MAKE THIS.

SERVES 4

2 courgettes weighing about 400g/14oz
1 tsp dried dill
6 large free range eggs
1 tsp olive oil
350g/12oz skinned and boned salmon
300ml/10 fl oz (½pt) natural Greek style unsweetened yoghurt
1 tsp cornflour
50g/1¾oz finely grated parmesan or other hard cheese
Salt and pepper to taste

You will need a 26cm/10 in non stick frying pan or chefs pan with a lid to make this.

Pre heat the oven to 200°C/ 400°F/Gas 5

Wash and dry the salmon and cut it into 1cm/½ in pieces.

Whisk one of the eggs, 1 tsp dried dill and 1 tsp cornflour into the yoghurt and put to one side.

Whisk the other 5 eggs in a large bowl and season to taste.

Coarsely grate the courgette and mix it into the eggs.

Heat the frying pan with 1 tsp olive oil over a medium heat and add the pieces of salmon. Cover and cook them in the oven for 5 minutes. By this time the fish should be just set and translucent. Use a slotted spoon to remove it from the pan and put it to one side.

Add the egg and courgette mixture to the pan and cook for 5 minutes over a moderate heat. Put on the lid and transfer the pan to the oven. Cook for 10 minutes.

Reduce the oven to 180°C/ 350°F/Gas 4

Take the frying pan out of the oven, remove the lid and put the salmon on top of the 'omelette' in a single layer. Pour the yoghurt and egg mixture on top. Put the pan back in the oven without the lid and bake for 10 minutes.

Pre heat the grill to high. Take the frying pan out of the oven, sprinkle on the grated cheese and pop it under the grill until the cheese has melted. Serve with green vegetables or a green salad.

Sardine Omelette

A STRANGE COMBINATION BUT ONE THAT TASTES REALLY GOOD AND IT IS QUICK AND EASY TO PREPARE. YOU CAN USE ANY TYPE OF TINNED OILY FISH TO MAKE THIS. SARDINES WORK PARTICULARLY WELL BUT MAKE SURE YOU USE SARDINE FILLETS THAT HAVE BEEN CANNED IN OLIVE OIL NOT SUNFLOWER OIL.

SERVES 2

120g/4¼ oz sardine fillets in olive oil
5 large free range eggs
4 spring onions sliced OR half red onion finely chopped
Half finely chopped red chilli or ½ tsp chilli paste
1 large or 2 small tomatoes finely sliced.
1 – 2 tbsp capers

Pour 1 tablespoon of the olive oil from the sardines into an omelette pan and optionally drain the rest away. Break up the sardine fillets into large flakes.

Whisk the eggs until the whites and yolks are combined. Stir in the onions, the chopped chilli or chilli paste and the sardines.

Heat the grill on high.

Heat the oil in the omelette pan over a medium heat and pour in the eggs, tipping the eggs from side to side so that they are evenly spread.

Using a fork gently draw the edges of the egg towards the centre of the pan and let the liquid egg run to the edges. Keep doing this until the omelette is almost set but still moist on top.

Turn off the heat and put a layer of sliced tomatoes over the top of the omelette. Put it under the grill for 2 – 3 minutes until the tomatoes are heated through. Serve immediately with some green vegetables or a green salad.

Tortilla, Frittata & Kuku

All of these have their origins in Kukus, a sort of solid unfolded omelette that contains vegetables and herbs. Kukus' originated in ancient Persia. It is hardly surprising that there is a similarity between the tortilla and the frittata as the kuku was brought to Spain by the Arabs and the spice traders brought it to Italy.

You can basically use more or less any vegetable to make kukus, tortillas and frittatas. Just make sure the ingredients are freshly cooked otherwise the finished dish will have a stale leftover taste. You can serve tortillas, frittatas and kukus hot or cold, as a main course, cut in slices for a picnic or cut into small squares as canapés. They make an excellent breakfast dish and they will keep for up to 2 days in a fridge.

Recipes for these types of egg dishes vary. Some add baking powder and some add flour, most are cooked slowly in a covered non stick frying pan. Whichever recipe you use and whichever way you choose to cook it, this type of egg dish provides a nutritious meal that is quick and easy to prepare.

Egg dishes of this type have a reputation of being a bit 'dried up'. Adding a small amount of cream, yoghurt or fromage frais helps prevent this. One thing you do need when making a tortilla, frittata or kuku is a high quality non stick frying pan, preferably one with a lid. If you can find one with a metal handle that you can put into the oven all the better as the easiest and fail safe way of cooking a tortilla or frittata is to start the process on the hob and then finish it in the oven.

Cauliflower, Tomato & Anchovy Frittata

THIS IS FRITTATA MAKES A SUBSTANTIAL FAMILY MEAL. YOU CAN EAT IT HOT, COLD OR AT ROOM TEMPERATURE. YOU WILL NEED A 24CM/10 IN NON STICK FRYING PAN WITH A LID TO MAKE THIS.

SERVES 4

6 large free range eggs
3 tbsp natural unsweetened yoghurt (optional)
2 cloves garlic crushed
1 tsp chilli paste, chilli flakes or Sambol Oelek
1 medium cauliflower broken into small florets
150g/5½oz cherry tomatoes cut in half
4 spring onions sliced
50g/1¾oz tin anchovy fillets
2 – 3 tbsp capers drained and rinsed
10 salted black olives, stones removed

Pre heat the oven to 180°C/ 350°F/Gas 4

Cook the cauliflower for 3 - 4 minutes. Drain and put to one side to cool a little.

Whisk the eggs in a large bowl with the Sambol Oelek, crushed garlic and yoghurt. Stir in the cauliflower, tomatoes, sliced spring onions, black olives and capers. Pour 1 tbsp of the olive oil from the anchovies into the frying pan and heat it over a medium heat. Pour in the egg and cauliflower mixture and cook for 5 minutes then cover it and put the pan into the oven. Cook for 20 minutes.

Pre heat the grill to high. Take the frying pan out of the oven, remove the lid and arrange the anchovy fillets on top. Pop it under the grill and cook for 3 – 4 minutes until the top of the tortilla is set and the anchovies have cooked through.

Broccoli & Red Pepper Tortilla

THIS TORTILLA IS BASED ON A SIMPLE ITALIAN WAY OF COOKING SPROUTING AND TENDER STEM BROCCOLI. THE ORIGINAL RECIPE USES 2 DRIED RED CHILLIES THAT ARE CRUSHED AND CRUMBLED INTO THE BROCCOLI. AS THIS CAN BE A BIT TOO HOT AND SPICY USING CHILLI POWDER, SAMBOL OELEK OR SOME OTHER FORM OF CHILLI PASTE ALLOWS YOU TO ADJUST THE 'HEAT' IN LINE WITH YOUR PALATE. BY ADDING EGGS AND YOGHURT AND SOME CHEESE THE BROCCOLI IS TRANSFORMED INTO A FAMILY MEAL OR SUBSTANTIAL BREAKFAST.

SERVES 4

500g/1lb 2oz broccoli, white or purple sprouting broccoli or sprouting kale.
2 tsp Sambol Oelek. OR chilli paste
1 large Ramiro pepper de-seeded and finely sliced into rings
4 spring onions sliced
10 dry salted black olives with stones removed
1 tbsp olive oil
100g/3½oz feta or goats cheese
6 large free range eggs
3 tbsp natural unsweetened yoghurt (optional)

You will need a 24cm/10 in non stick frying pan or chefs pan with a lid to make this. Pre heat the oven to 180°C/350°F/Gas 4

Heat 1 tablespoon of the olive oil in a the frying pan. Add the red pepper and cook over a medium heat for 5 minutes to extract the flavour from the peppers. Turn the heat to low while you cook the broccoli.

Trim off any tough stalks and leaves from the broccoli. If the stems are thick cut them off and then cut them in half lengthways. Bring a large pan of water to the boil. Add the broccoli, bring it back to the boil and cook for 2 to 3 minutes until just tender. Drain and add it to the red peppers.

Whisk the eggs in a large bowl with the Sambol Oelek and yoghurt. Stir in the sliced spring onions and black olives.

Mix the broccoli and peppers together and pour in the egg mixture over them. Cook for 5 minutes then cover the frying pan and put it into the oven. Cook for 20 minutes. Take off the lid and cook for another 5 minutes until the centre of the tortilla is just set.

Tofu, Bean Curd & Tempeh

Soy beans in the form of tofu, bean curd and Tempeh are healthy high protein foods, but when they come in the form of 'imitation' meat or when soy bean is added as 'textured vegetable protein' to make vegie burgers, pad out processed meat products and make junk food like soya cheese and ice cream they are far from healthy.

The soya used to make textured vegetable protein and soya cheese and ice cream is usually a bye-product of the manufacture of soya bean oil and as a result it is very heavily processed. In addition these types of soy bean products are often made from genetically modified soya bean crops and the jury is still out on whether or not these are safe to eat.

Why?

Tofu, bean curd and Tempeh, which is also called bean cake, are amazing products that have been staple foods in China, Japan and the Far East for thousands of years. They are high in protein and contain all of the essential amino acids. As well as being low in fat, low in calories, easy to digest and cheap, they also contain high levels of vitamin A and the B vitamins. They are all an excellent source of iron, calcium, manganese, selenium, copper, zinc and magnesium. Tempeh is particularly rich in vitamin B12 which is rare in vegetable products and gram for gram it contains the same amount of protein as meat. A hundred grams of Tempeh provides between 35% and 40% of an adults recommended daily intake of protein.

Tofu in the form of bean curd originated in China over one thousand years ago. Originally it was the poor man's protein but when one of the Emperors started eating it it became fashionable and soon it was more or less a staple food. It has remained so ever since.

Tofu and bean curd are 'processed' products. They are made from dried soya beans in a process that is fairly similar to cheese making. The soya beans used can be black, green or white and this is sometimes reflected in the colour of the tofu. The whole beans are soaked and then ground into a thick paste that is then boiled. The fluid is drained off and a coagulant is then added. The solid 'curds' are separated out and then pressed into blocks. Even though tofu and bean curd are processed foods they are very close to the dried soya beans they are made from. If you look at the label you will see soya beans, water and in the case of bean curd, coagulants such as calcium sulphite (gypsum), nigari (magnesium chlorate) or GDL (delta glucano lactose). They may sound horrendous but these coagulants have been used to make the product for hundreds of years.

Tempeh is thought to have originated in Indonesia in the 12th or 13th century. The Chinese had introduced tofu making there and the story is that some soaked soy beans that had been left uncovered became contaminated with some spores that grew a fungus that was found to be edible. Adding a natural live mould culture to soy beans that have been soaked, de-skinned and partially cooked is all that is needed to make Tempeh. After the culture is added the beans are spread on trays in a thin layer and left to ferment for twenty four to thirty six hours in a warm environment. The mould grows and knits the beans together into a 'cake'. Hence the name bean cake.

Are soy bean products safe to eat?

There is currently a lot of controversy about whether tofu, bean curd, Tempeh and soya bean products in general are safe to eat. If you do an internet search using "tofu and health" you will be bombarded by a raft of information telling how harmful and dangerous they are. Are they as bad as people make out? After all they are foods that have been consumed by people in the Far East for thousands of years and most of the people who eat them today are far healthier than their Western counterparts. The Okinawans in Japan are some of the world's healthiest and long lived people and, together with fish, tofu is one of their staple foods.

One of the most frequently used arguments about tofu, bean curd and Tempeh is that the soy beans they are made from contain large amounts of toxins and anti-nutrients which can give rise to a variety of gastric problems and nutrient deficiencies. The three main anti-nutrients in soy beans are trypsin inhibitors, phytates and lectins. These are the same anti-nutrients that are found in grains and in varying amounts in nuts and more or less all vegetables, fruit and pulses. Everyone agrees that eating raw soy beans is not a good idea. However, soaking and then cooking the soy beans before they are made into tofu tends to deactivate some of the trypsin inhibitors and eliminate a good amount of the phytates and lectins. Because Tempeh is fermented most if not all of the trypsin inhibitors and phytates are removed during the fermentation process. So just like grains, cereals, pulses and vegetables soy bean products do contain some anti-nutrients but when you look at the big picture unless you consume them in enormous amounts they are unlikely to pose a threat to your well being.

Another argument that is often used as a reason for not eating tofu is that tofu is to blame for a 'lazy' thyroid. This is because soy beans contain high levels of compounds called goitrogens which are known to disrupt the production of thyroid hormones. So any soy bean product, tofu, bean curd and Tempeh, are bound to have a damaging effect on your metabolism. Well do they? Like many other food scares this starts out from some sort of truth. Soy beans and soy bean products do have the potential to affect your thyroid gland but so do all the other vegetables that contain goitrogens. Vegetables like broccoli, cauliflower, cabbage, kales and Brussel sprouts. It is a very long list. So it is unlikely that eating tofu, bean curd or Tempeh will cause thyroid problems in healthy people. The exception is people with a diagnosed thyroid problem or people with a very low intake of iodine. So the solution is to consume tofu, bean curd and Tempeh with small amounts of seaweed or other iodine rich foods, like cod, bananas, cranberries, unpasteurised dairy products, strawberries and whole grain cereals. In other words as part of a healthy diet.

Irrespective of its nutritional content, one really important reason why Tempeh in particular should feature on your menu is that it is a fermented food and fermented foods are known to nourish the healthy bacteria in your digestive tract and this will help boost your immune system.

How

You will find fresh tofu and bean curd in Asian food stores and most supermarkets now stock pasteurised 'long life' brands. Until fairly recently Tempeh was much more difficult to obtain but with increasing interest in fermented foods Tempeh is now becoming more widely available and because it freezes extremely well the easiest source of supply is to buy it frozen on the internet.

Tempeh has a firm 'meaty' texture while tofu comes in different textures, from firm down to 'silken'. Together they are a major source of protein to committed vegetarians and vegans. To others tofu in particular is 'Terrible Tofu', 'Tasteless Tofu' or 'Rubbery squares that look awful'. You rarely hear a good word said about it. However, what it looks like and what it tastes like depend on how it is cooked and one of the great things about soya bean products in general is that they absorb the flavours of the things that they are cooked with.

Tofu, bean curd and Tempeh can be steamed, poached in a sauce, lightly sautéed, crumbled into vegetables and even puréed to make dips and salad dressings. Dare I say it, but they can also be marinated and then roasted, baked or fried. Silken tofu makes really good 'cheesecakes' and it provides a highly nutritious base for terrines. It is particularly valuable for people who are lactose intolerant as it can be used as a substitute for cream and yogurt.

Tofu with Scrambled Egg & Chilli

THIS IS ONE OF THOSE SUPER QUICK MEALS THAT YOU CAN HAVE READY IN MINUTES. YOU WILL NEED FIRM TOFU OR TEMPEH TO MAKE THIS.

SERVES 4

2 tsp finely grated lemon zest
1 tbsp light soy sauce
1 tbsp rice vinegar
1 tbsp lemon juice
1 tsp sugar
1 clove garlic crushed
250g/9oz firm tofu
1 tbsp fine polenta for dusting
1 tbsp olive oil
1 red chilli finely sliced OR 1tsp Sambol Oelek
1 red pepper finely diced
4 large free range eggs beaten
sliced red chilli or red pepper to garnish.

Combine the lemon zest, light soy sauce, rice vinegar, lemon juice and sugar in a bowl.

Cut the tofu into bite size pieces about 1cm/½in thick. Marinade it in the lemon and soy mixture for half an hour. Take the tofu out of the marinade and put the marinade to one side. Dry the tofu and lightly dust it with polenta.

Heat the oil in a wok or frying pan and cook the tofu over a medium heat to seal it.

Remove the tofu from the pan and add the red pepper and chilli. Stir fry for 2 minutes, then add the crushed garlic, keeping everything moving so that the garlic does not go brown and burn.

Add the marinade mixture, stir and add the beaten eggs and the tofu.

Reduce the heat and cook very slowly until the eggs are just set. Garnish with finely sliced red chilli or red pepper before serving.

Vegetable Torte

A PASTRY-LESS QUICHE. THAT YOU CAN MAKE IT WITH MORE OR LESS ANY VEGETABLES THAT YOU HAVE AVAILABLE. THE TORTE WILL KEEP FOR UP TO 2 DAYS IN THE FRIDGE BUT IT WILL NOT FREEZE.

SERVES 6 - 8

250g/9oz courgettes
250g/9oz cauliflower broken into small florets
70g/2½oz fine French beans
1 medium white onion finely chopped
1 tbsp olive oil
2 cloves of garlic crushed
2 finely chopped preserved lemons
2 tbsp chopped basil
5 tbsp finely grated parmesan
200g/7oz feta
350g/12oz silken tofu
4 large free range eggs

Pre heat the oven to 160°C/325°F/Gas 3

Grease a 20cm/8 in cake tin and dust the inside with finely grated parmesan.

Sauté the onion and garlic in the olive oil over a medium heat for 5 minutes. Stir it occasionally, do not let it brown. Put them to one side.

Top and tail the French beans. Add them to a pan of boiling water and cook them for 3 – 4 minutes. Drain and refresh them in cold water.

Put the cauliflower into a large microwave bowl, add 3 tablespoons of water, cover and cook on full power for 3 minutes. Take the cauliflower out and put it to one side.

If the courgettes are large cut them in half lengthways and cut each half into 5mm/¼ in slices.

Put the sliced courgette and the mange tout into the microwave bowl, cover and cook for 3 minutes. Leave to cool.

Cut half of the feta into small 5mm/¼ in dice. Put the rest into a bowl with the tofu, eggs, chopped basil and the parmesan and blend everything together using a hand blender.

Stir in the onions, the vegetables, the chopped preserved lemons and diced feta.

Pour the mixture into the prepared cake tin, cover loosely with foil and bake in the centre of the oven for 45 minutes. Take the foil off and cook for another 15 minutes. Turn off the oven and leave the torte to cool before taking it out.

Carrot, Lentil & Pistachio Loaf

THIS RECIPE USES SILKEN TOFU TO ADD ADDITIONAL PROTEIN TO THE LENTILS. THE LOAF MAKES A SUBSTANTIAL FAMILY MEAL. IT CAN BE MADE IN ADVANCE, COOKED AND THEN WARMED UP WHEN NEEDED. IT DOES NOT FREEZE WELL ONCE IT IS COOKED BUT IT CAN BE FROZEN UNCOOKED.

SERVES 4 - 6

1 large free range egg
50g/1½oz finely chopped coriander OR
30g/1oz coriander pesto
2 tbsp grated ginger
200g/6½oz red lentils
400g/13oz carrots, peeled and finely grated
50g/1½oz shelled pistachio nuts
350g/12oz silken tofu
1 clove garlic crushed (optional)

Grease and line a 1.4Lt/2 ½ pt loaf tin and heat the oven to 180°C/ 350°F/Gas 4.

Wash the lentils and pick them over carefully to make sure there is no grit in them. Drain them in a sieve, put them into a saucepan and add 350ml/12 fl oz of cold water. Bring them to the boil, cover, turn down the heat to low and cook very slowly for 20 minutes. The lentils should be just cooked and the water absorbed. Leave them to cool a little.

Put the grated carrot and the grated ginger into a microwave bowl. Cover and cook on full power for 5 minutes. Take off the cover and leave to cool a little.

Drain the tofu and put it into a large bowl with the egg. Use a hand blender to blend it thoroughly into a thick paste.

Add the grated carrot, the cooked lentils, the garlic, pistachio nuts and the chopped coriander to the tofu and egg mixture. Give it a good stir and put it into the loaf tin and bake for half an hour. Turn the oven down to 160°C/ 325°F/Gas 3 and bake for another 30 minutes. Leave for 5 to 10 minutes before serving.

Tempeh with Ginger, Chilli & Leeks

YOU CAN USE TEMPEH, FIRM TOFU OR THE MICRO PROTEIN QUORN. UNLIKE TOFU TEMPEH FREEZES AND WHILE FRESH TEMPEH IS DIFFICULT TO OBTAIN, FROZEN TEMPEH IS READILY AVAILABLE.

SERVES 4

225g/8oz Tempeh cut into ½cm/¼in slices
2 tbsp olive oil
1 tsp sesame oil
1 tsp Sambol Oelek or 1 finely chopped red chilli
1 tbsp finely grated ginger
2 tbsp light soy sauce
1tbsp dry sherry or vermouth
3 leeks, white only, finely sliced
1 small Ramiro pepper finely sliced
50ml/5 fl oz vegetable stock
1 tbsp cornflour

Mix the grated ginger, Sambol Oelek, soy sauce, sherry and sesame oil together in a bowl. Add the slices of Tempeh stir them around and leave them to marinade for 30 minutes.

Strain the Tempeh from the marinade but keep the marinade. Add the stock, and the cornflour to the marinade to make a paste.

Heat the oil in a wok or large frying pan and sauté the Tempeh until it is lightly browned. Remove it and put to one side.

Sauté the leeks and Ramiro pepper for 4 – 5 minutes until the leeks are tender. Return the Tempeh to the pan together with the marinade and cornflour mixture and stir well until the liquid becomes clear.

Fermented foods

In the form of Miso, Kefir, Sauerkraut, Kimchee, Natto and cheese made from raw unpasteurized milk.

Why?

When foods are fermented the fermentation process 'pre digests' them and this makes it easier for us to digest them and absorb the nutrients that they contain. Fermented foods are excellent sources of protein, vitamins and minerals and they play an important role in helping us build and maintain a healthy population of bacteria in our digestive tract. Most of us who are eating a conventional Western diet do not have a healthy population of bacteria so eating prebiotic foods that support the growth of them is one of the best things we can do. Foods rich in resistant starch and soluble and insoluble fibre are key to this but fermented foods are brimming with the bacteria that are needed to build and maintain a healthy population.

Fermentation has been used as a method of preserving food for thousands of years and as a consequence there are hundreds of different fermented foods around the world. The six that are most readily available and easy to use are Miso, Kefir, Sauerkraut, Kimchee, Natto and cheese that is made from raw milk.

Miso

Miso is one of the best loved and easy to use fermented food. It gives food a deep salty, savoury, slightly sweet flavour. It forms a staple part of the diet in Japan and Korea and to a lesser extent in China. Miso is made by fermenting soy bean, barley or brown rice with a fungus called koji. The end result of the fermentation process is a paste that comes in colours ranging from brown or red through to yellow and white. The darker the color the stronger the flavour.

Kefir

Kefir is a fermented milk product that originated in Russia and the Balkans. It can be made from any type of cow, goat or sheep milk and it is now becoming widely available made from coconut milk. It is slightly acid and tastes like a drinkable 'live' yogurt. As well as plenty of live healthy bacteria, it also contains vitamin B12 and vitamin K2.

Kefir is easy to make at home. It is made from grains that resemble miniature cauliflower florets and you can buy these on the internet. Once the kefir culture is started you can go on using it to make more kefir in much the same way as you do when making your own yogurt. Ready to drink Kefir is becoming widely available in supermarkets but check the label carefully is it sometimes contains added sugar and flavouring.

Sauerkraut

Sauerkraut is an old traditional food that is made from white cabbage that has been finely sliced, lightly salted and then fermented by various naturally occurring bacteria. It is packed full of vitamins and dietary fibre. Just 100g of sauerkraut contains 24% of your daily requirement for vitamin C and 11% of your daily requirement for dietary fibre.

Kimchee

Kimchee is a traditional Korean food that dates back to the 7th century. Most Koreans eat it at least once a day. It is made by salting and fermenting vegetables. The most widely found Kimchee is made from cabbage, usually Napa cabbage or Chinese leaf, that is salted, rinsed and then mixed with other vegetables like Korean radish and onions. Ginger, chilli and garlic are added and the Kimchee is then left to ferment for several days. Traditional Kimchee has quite a strong flavour that some people may find unpleasant. Because of the interest in pro and pre biotic foods it is becoming more widely available outside of Asian food stores but it is also easy to make, both as authentic Kimchee or as a 'quick' alternative. If you look on the internet you will find plenty of sites, each with their own recipes.

Natto

Natto is a popular food in Japan that is usually eaten with boiled rice. Like Tempeh it is made from fermented soy beans, but unlike Tempeh it has a slimy texture and a very strong smell that is reminiscent of ripe unpasteurized cheese. As a result it is not to everyone's taste. It is however a very powerful prebiotic and it contains a powerful anti-inflammatory enzyme called nattokinase.

Unpasteurized cheese

Cheese that has been made from raw cow, goat or sheep milk. Up until only fairly recent history more or less all cheese was made from raw milk but with the change from cottage industry to large commercial scale manufacturing more and more cheese was made from pasteurized milk. As a result unpasteurized cheese was difficult to find. With the growing interest in artisan cheeses and pre and probiotic foods, unpasteurized cheese is now becoming more widely available. Like some other fermented foods cheese made from raw milk is often covered in a mould and it usually has a strong smell and a strong taste.

If you eat unpasteurized cheese and dairy products Listeria is something you need to be aware of. Healthy adults occasionally become infected with Listeria but they rarely become seriously ill. However, just about all health authorities recommend that pregnant women, young children, the elderly and people with a compromised immune system do not eat this type of cheese as it does pose a risk to their health.

How

If you are new to fermented foods start with a small portion, around half a cup a day and gradually build up the amount you are eating over a week or two. When you are using Miso add it to the dish at the last minute in order to preserve its flavour and nutritional value. Miso can be used to make excellent soup as well as dips and marinades for meat and fish.

For many of us who have been eating a conventional Western diet the taste of some fermented food can be quite strong, it is something of an acquired taste. In the case of unpasteurized cheese this is a bonus as you need far less cheese to provide an acceptable flavour and satisfy your appetite.

Miso, Tofu & Tahini Dip with Crudités

SILKEN TOFU CAN BE MADE INTO DIPS AND IT IS A VERY USEFUL INGREDIENT FOR PEOPLE WHO ARE UNABLE TO EAT DAIRY PRODUCTS. THIS IS AN INTERESTING DIP THAT CAN BE SERVED ON ITS OWN, WITH CRUDITÉS OR USED AS A DRESSING FOR VEGETABLES AND NOODLES. IT FREEZES WELL BUT LEAVE OUT THE GARLIC IF YOU ARE GOING TO FREEZE IT AND ADD IT LATER.

350g/12oz silken tofu
2 cloves garlic crushed
2 tbsp white miso
8 tbsp Tahini
Juice of 1 lemon OR 2 limes
3 tbsp light soy sauce
Crushed black pepper to taste
4 tbsp finely sliced chives

Put everything together in a bowl and blend with a hand blender until you have a smooth paste. Stir in half of the chives, put the dip into a serving bowl and sprinkle the remaining chives on top.

Uppingham Pâté

THIS IS A RECIPE FOR USING UP OLD BLUE STILTON CHEESE. MATURE BLUE STILTON MAKES THE BEST UPPINGHAM PÂTÉ BUT YOU CAN USE ANY TYPE OF BLUE CHEESE. SERVE IT WITH BABY BEETROOT, SOME SALAD LEAVES AND A HANDFUL OF WALNUTS OR AS A DIP WITH CRUDITÉS. IT. THE PÂTÉ CAN BE KEPT IN THE FRIDGE FOR 4 TO 5 DAYS. IT CAN ALSO BE FROZEN FOR 1 TO 2 MONTHS.

700ml/25 fl oz/1¼pt milk
1 large onion roughly chopped
1 large carrot peeled and roughly chopped
2 stalks celery chopped
1 tsp dried mixed herbs
85g/3oz butter
85g/3oz flour
2 tbsp lemon juice
1 - 2 cloves garlic crushed
15 stoned green olives finely chopped
½ tsp salt
½ tsp black pepper
¼ – ½ tsp cayenne pepper
350g/12oz Stilton cheese rind removed and crumbled

Put the milk into a saucepan and add the onion, carrot, celery and mixed herbs. Bring to the boil, reduce the heat and simmer uncovered for 20 minutes.

Remove from the heat and leave it to cool a little. Strain the milk through a sieve into a large bowl, pressing with a wooden spoon to extract as much juice as possible from the vegetables. Discard the contents of the sieve and set the milk to one side.

Melt the butter in a saucepan over a medium heat. Whisk in the flour and cook for 2 minutes stirring constantly. Slowly whisk in the milk and cook until the sauce is thick and smooth. Turn the heat to very low and let the sauce cook for 5 minutes. Set the sauce aside to cool.

When the sauce is cool add the cheese, lemon juice, crushed garlic, salt pepper and cayenne. Use a hand blender to blend it until it is smooth, then stir in the chopped olives. Cover with cling film and chill for at least an hour before serving.

Butter and Other Saturated Fats

Why?

It is a fact that any fat or oil can become harmful when it is oxidised. The more saturated a fat is the less likely it is to oxidise. The first big food fib was that saturated fats were bad for us so we stopped eating them. This had the effect of over loading our bodies with vegetable oils that oxidised and depriving our bodies of healthy saturated fats that did not oxidise. The oxidised vegetable oils damaged our health and because the saturated fats were needed to repair damaged cells and help build hormones, enzymes, Vitamin D and some of our body's antioxidant defences our health suffered even more.

With the exception of people who are genetically predisposed to developing high levels of cholesterol, it is perfectly safe for us to consume saturated fat, provided it forms part of a healthy diet that includes plenty of vegetables. Like eggs, butter has been part of our diet for thousands of years and the saturated fat it contains is not in itself bad. It is the consumption of sugar, over refined carbohydrates, chemically altered foods and a lack of antioxidants, vitamins and minerals that is making us ill. It is an interesting fact that in the UK we each eat 1.4Kg of flour a week but only 39 grams of butter.

How?

Eat and enjoy but in moderation. Eat only pure butter, not spreadable homogenised butter or butter that is mixed with vegetable oils and trans fats. Remember, fat is a high energy food. One gram of fat contains about 9kcals of energy. One gram of carbohydrate contains about 4kcal. However, because it takes longer to digest, fat will make you feel full for much longer than carbohydrate, especially if the carbohydrate is highly refined. Use a teaspoon as a means of portion control. You will be surprised to learn that one teaspoon contains about 8 grams of butter and as butter is 80% fat this amounts to 50 calories a teaspoon, so be mindful of how much you use. Where ever you use margarine replace it with butter. Butter oxidises far less than polyunsaturated oils when it is heated but irrespective of what type of fat you use fried foods are not a particularly healthy option.

Are there other saturated fats?

A clarified form of butter called ghee has been used for cooking in India for centuries. Interestingly as it contains virtually no lactose it is fine for people who are otherwise lactose intolerant. It has a slightly nutty flavour and you can usually find it in Asian food stores. Also goose fat and dare I say it coconut oil and things like lard are making a comeback.

What about the Omega 6 polyunsaturated oils in lard and goose fat? Well some people think that it is bad but in reality it needs to be put into perspective as the amount of Omega 6 in them is not very different to the amount found in olive oil and it is far less than the amount of Omega 6 found in polyunsaturated vegetable oils.

The bottom line is that our bodies need saturated fats. We just need to remember that like all fats and oils they are high in calories and should be eaten in moderate amounts as part of a balanced diet that includes plenty of vegetables.

Olives & Olive Oil

Why?

Olive oil is a monounsaturated fat that has been around for a very long time. It contains large amounts of oleic acid and this is the most commonly found monounsaturated fatty acid in our bodies. Oleic acid is also found in oils from almonds, pecans, cashews, peanuts and avocados.

Olive oil contains 75% oleic acid, 13% saturated fat in the form of palmitic acid, 10% Omega 6 and 2% Omega 3. Despite the five to one ratio of Omega 6 to Omega 3 the large amount of monounsaturated fatty acids makes it a very healthy oil. It is also rich in phytonutrients that have antioxidant, anti-inflammatory and anti-bacterial properties. Olive oil is an oil that has been widely used in Mediterranean, North African and Middle Eastern cooking for thousands of years and it has withstood the test of time. There is no doubt that it is the safest vegetable oil you can use, provided of course that it is consumed in sensible amounts. At the end of the day olive oil is a fat. One gram weighs in so to speak at just under 9kcal, so for a teaspoon think 40kcal and for a tablespoon think 120kcal.

Like olive oil, olives have been around for thousands of years. In the west most of us eat them as a snack but in Mediterranean and North African countries they are part of people's staple diet. Some olives are green and some are black. Some are preserved in oil and some are preserved in brine. Some come in jars and some come in cans. Green olives have a very different taste to black olives, and some black olives have a metallic taste.

So what is the difference between green olives and black olives and is one better to eat than the other? Green olives are picked before they are ripe and black olives are picked when they are ripe. When they are first picked all olives are bitter and inedible so they go through a curing process that involves soaking them in water for a week or two and then pickling them in brine. Green olives need to be kept in brine for three months and black olives for nine months. They are then ready to eat or for marinading in oil and storing in jars.

The length of time it takes to process olives means they often go through a fast curing process that involves adding caustic soda, E524, to the soaking water and then pasteurising or sterilising the olives to kill bacteria. When you buy black olives that have gone through the fast process they are in fact green olives that have been dyed with ferrous gluconate, E579. This gives the olives a uniform black colour but it also gives them a metallic taste. Because it is part of the curing process you will not see caustic soda on the label but if the olives have been dyed the label should declare ferrous gluconate or E579. As a general rule tinned brined olives are most likely to have gone though the fast process so the best advice is to go for olives marinaded in olive oil and sold in jars.

How?

Keep olive oil in a dark bottle or in the fridge. Simply use it everywhere you would otherwise have used polyunsaturated oils but do not deep fat fry food with it. Instead lightly sauté your food or bake it a moderate temperature. Olive oil also makes great salad dressings mixed with lemon juice, vinegar and herbs.

Tapenade

AN OLIVE PURÉE THAT YOU CAN MAKE WITH EITHER BLACK OR GREEN OLIVES. IF YOU ARE USING BLACK OLIVES TRY TO OBTAIN THE DRY SALTED ONES FROM TURKEY OR MOROCCO AS THEY HAVE A MUCH FINER FLAVOUR AND THEY ARE LESS LIKELY TO HAVE BEEN DYED.

85g/3oz pitted black olives
4 anchovy fillets OR 2 tsp anchovy paste
35g/1¼oz capers
2 cloves garlic crushed or more or less to taste
4 tbsp olive oil
½ finely chopped red chilli (optional)

If the olives have been salted soak them overnight.

Put everything into a blender or food processor and blitz until you have a smooth but slightly grainy paste.

Olive & Anchovy Bites

WITH THE ANCHOVIES AND CAYENNE PEPPER THESE MELT IN THE MOUTH BISCUITS ARE A HEALTHY TREAT. THEY STORE VERY WELL AND CAN BE KEPT IN AN AIRTIGHT CONTAINER IN THE FRIDGE FOR UP TO 2 WEEKS. YOU CAN ALSO FREEZE THEM FOR UP TO 3 MONTHS.

Makes a 40 – 45
175g/6oz whole grain spelt
1 tsp cayenne pepper
50g/1¾oz butter
4 tbsp finely grated parmesan
50g/1¾oz tin anchovy fillets in olive oil roughly chopped
50g/1¾oz chopped salted black olives

Place all of the ingredients except the black olives into a food processor and pulse until the mixture forms a firm dough.

Put the dough onto a piece of baking parchment and knead in the chopped olives. Wrap the dough in cling film and chill for half an hour.

Pre heat the oven to 200°C/ 400°F/Gas 5 and line 2 large baking trays with baking parchment or non stick foil.

Put the dough onto a sheet of lightly floured baking parchment or cling film. Cover with another sheet of baking parchment or cling film and roll it until it is 3 – 4 mm thick.

Cut it into strips 5cm/2 in wide. Then cut each strip diagonally in alternative directions to make triangles.

Put the biscuits onto the baking trays and bake for 8 – 10 minutes until they are golden brown. Cool on a wire rack.

Olive & Almond Spread

THIS IS A RICH AND CONCENTRATED SPREAD THAT IS IN BETWEEN A PESTO AND A TAPENADE. IN TERMS OF FLAVOUR A LITTLE GOES A LONG WAY.

100g/3½oz pitted black olives
100g/3½oz ground almonds
1 tbsp capers
1 tbsp olive oil
Crushed garlic (optional)
1 tsp Sambol Oelek

Put everything into a blender and blend into a purée. Add a little water if the mixture looks too dry.

Pizza with Onions, Anchovies & Olives

NOT QUITE THE PIZZA WE ARE USED TO BUT JUST AS GOOD AND IT IS MUCH QUICKER TO MAKE AS THERE IS NO NEED TO PROVE THE DOUGH OR ROLL OUT THE BASE. THE PIZZA 'CRUST' IS AN ADAPTATION OF AN 18TH CENTURY RECIPE FOR SODA BREAD.

YOU CAN MAKE THE PIZZA BASE AND USE ANY TYPE OF TOPPING, WITH OR WITHOUT TOMATO AND WITH OR WITHOUT CHEESE. THIS RECIPE USES JUST ONIONS, ANCHOVIES AND OLIVES. BOTH THE PIZZA BASE AND THE ONION CONFIT USED AS THE TOPPING CAN BE MADE IN ADVANCE AND STORED IN THE FRIDGE. BOTH OF THEM FREEZE WELL.

SERVES 4

FOR THE PIZZA BASE
½ cup wholegrain spelt
½ cup fine oatmeal
1 tsp baking powder
3 tbsp olive oil
1 cup milk
¼ cup milk

FOR THE TOPPING
450g/1lb white onions finely sliced
100g/3½oz soft low fat cheese such as Quark or ricotta
Finely grated zest of ½ lemon
Juice of ½ lemon
2 bay leaves
Crushed black pepper
50g/1¾oz tin anchovy fillets in olive oil
24 salted black olives stones removed and cut in half
2 tbsp pine nuts (optional)

You will need a 24cm/10 in round silicon tin or spring form tin to make this. If you are using an ordinary tin grease it well.

First put 1 cup of milk into a bowl and whisk in the olive oil. Then stir in the fine oatmeal. Leave the oatmeal to soak while you prepare the onion confit.

Drain half of the oil from the anchovies into a saucepan, add the onions and gently sauté them over a medium heat for 5 minutes.

Add the bay leaves and lemon zest, cover the saucepan, reduce the heat to very low and simmer the onions for 30 – 40 minutes until they are soft. Check them once in a while to make sure that they are not sticking or turning brown. Add a tablespoon of water if you need to.

Remove the bay leaves and leave the onions to cool slightly before stirring in the lemon juice and the ricotta.

Pre heat the oven to 200°C/ 400°F/Gas 5

To make the pizza base. Stir ¼ cup of milk into the soaked oatmeal. Mix the spelt, and baking powder together and add this to the oatmeal. It will start bubbling as soon as the flour is added so mix it quickly to form a batter and pour it into the baking tin. Put it into the oven straight away and bake for 12 minutes. By this time it should be lightly browned and firm to the touch. Turn it over and put it back into the oven for 3 minutes to dry off the base.

To assemble the pizza, put the pizza base onto an ovenproof plate or baking tray and spoon on the onion mixture. Arrange the black olives and anchovies on top and sprinkle on the pine nuts if you are using them. Drizzle over the remaining oil from the anchovy fillets. Bake for 10 minutes to heat the topping through and lightly toast the pine nuts.

Aubergine Melanzane

ONE OF THE DELIGHTS OF ITALIAN COOKING THAT HAS FOUND ITS WAY AROUND THE WORLD. MELANZANE BENEFITS FROM BEING COOKED AND THEN REHEATED AS THIS ALLOWS THE FLAVOURS TO DEVELOP. THE ANCHOVIES ARE AN OPTIONAL ADDITION. MELANZANE FREEZES VERY WELL. SERVE IT WITH A SIMPLE GREEN SALAD OR SOME GREEN VEGETABLES.

SERVES 4

1½ kg/3lbs Aubergine
2 tbsp olive oil (or the oil from the tin of anchovies)
500ml/18fl oz Passata (sieved tomato)
3 tbsp Tomato purée
2 tsp vegetable stock powder
250g/8oz) Mozzarella or Feta
2 - 3 cloves of garli3 - crushed
Finely grated parmesan
Large handful of basil leaves
4 tbsp black olives cut in half and stones removed
80g Tin anchovy fillets in olive oil (optional)

Pre heat the oven to 180°C/ 350°F/Gas 4

Slice the aubergines about 5mm/¼in thick. Put them into a microwave bowl, cover and microwave on full power for about 5 minutes until they are soft.

Heat the Passata, stir in the tomato concentrate, the bouillon powder, the crushed garlic and the oil. Leave to simmer on a low heat for about 10 minutes.

Grease a wide shallow ovenproof dish or tin. Put a layer of the cooked aubergine over the base, then add some tomato sauce, some torn basil leaves, olives or capers, some of the cheese and a scatter of parmesan.

Add another layer of aubergine, tomato sauce, basil, cheese and olives and finish with a layer of tomato.

Tear up the anchovy fillets and scatter them over the top. Bake for 45 minutes.

Water; good old fashioned 'Adams Ale'

Why?

Many of us do not drink enough water, or to be more precise, we do not drink the amount of water we individually need, and that could well be entirely different to the amount somebody else needs to drink.

When you read about drinking water, eight glasses a day keeps cropping up. Where this figure comes from is anyone's guess, but you do need to keep yourself well hydrated. We know that our body is 60% water and that we lose around forty fluid ounces or just over a litre of water a day, but this amount increases dramatically when we are exercising or in a hot environment. You will learn by trial and error how much you as an individual need to drink. The bottom line is that your urine needs to be light in colour and clear. The quality of tap water varies tremendously so it is up to you whether you buy bottled water or invest in a water filter or water purifier.

Tip:

Put soup onto the menu. In fact put it at the top of the menu. Soup as part of your meal will help hydrate you and because it helps to fill you up you will probably eat less. Remember coffee and alcohol dehydrate you so take a glass of water with your coffee or glass of wine. If you are bored with water make your own lemonade from lemons or limes. It freezes well and you can add dried elder flowers and black currents for variety. Last but not least remember to drink plenty of green, white or oolong tea.

Gazpacho

THIS SUMMER SOUP NEEDS NO COOKING. YOU CAN PREPARE IT IN ADVANCE AND KEEP IT FOR UP TO 24 HOURS IN THE FRIDGE.

SERVES 4

1 medium red onion
1 red or green pepper de-seeded
½ large telegraph cucumber
500g/1 lb ripe vine tomatoes
60g/2oz stale white bread
2 cloves of garlic crushed
2tbsp red wine vinegar
2tbsp olive oil
salt and freshly ground black pepper
1 large tomato to garnish
To Serve
Tabasco, Tahini and basil pesto

First you need to peel the tomatoes. Put them in a bowl and cover them with boiling water. Leave them for about a minute and then plunge them into ice cold water. The skins will have split and they will peel off quite easily.

Cut the onion, pepper and cucumber into large chunks. Put them into a food processor or blender and process them for a few seconds. Try to keep the texture fairly chunky. Transfer a quarter of the chopped vegetables to a bowl, cover the bowl and refrigerate. These vegetables will be used later as a garnish.

Add the tomatoes, bread, garlic vinegar and olive oil to the remainder of the vegetables in the food processor and blend once more. If the soup looks a little thick add some cold water. Season with salt and pepper, cover and place in the fridge to chill.

When you are ready to serve the soup finely chop the remaining tomato and add it to the bowl of reserved vegetables. Ladle the soup into a large serving bowl. Serve the vegetables in a separate bowl with some Tabasco and basil pesto.

Ginger, Noodle & Mushroom Soup

THIS RECIPE USES SOBA NOODLES THAT ARE MADE FROM BUCKWHEAT BUT YOU CAN USE ANY TYPE OF EGG OR RICE NOODLES. IF YOU USE DRIED SHITAKE MUSHROOMS FOLLOW THE REHYDRATION AND COOKING INSTRUCTIONS ON THE PACKET.

SERVES 4

200g/7oz chestnut mushrooms cut into 5mm/¼ in slices OR 15g/½oz dried shitake mushrooms
1Lt/1¾ pt/35 fl oz vegetable stock

Bring a saucepan of water to the boil. Add the soba noodles and cook following the instructions on the packet. This is usually about 8 minutes. Drain and stir in a small amount of olive oil to stop the noodles sticking together. Put them to one side while you cook the

125g/4½ oz soba noodles
2 tbsp olive oil
3 cloves of garlic finely chopped
1 tsp Sambol Oelek or ½ tsp chilli powder
2 tbsp grated ginger
1 tsp light soy sauce
125g/4½oz bean sprouts washed and drained OR finely sliced Chinese leaf
Roughly chopped coriander to garnish

mushrooms.

Heat the oil in a saucepan and sauté the mushrooms over a medium heat for 2 to 3 minutes. Add the garlic and ginger and cook for another 2 minutes.

Add the vegetable stock, the chilli and soy sauce and bring to the boil. Add the bean sprouts and bring the stock back to the boil, then add the cooked noodles and heat them through.

Serve garnished with the coriander.

Hot & Sour Soup With Watercress

A VERY EASY SOUP THAT YOU CAN HAVE READY IN MINUTES. YOU CAN USE ANY TYPE OF MUSHROOM INCLUDING DRIED MUSHROOMS. TAMARIND HAS A UNIQUE TART SLIGHTLY SOUR FLAVOUR AND IS WIDELY USED IN ASIAN COOKING. IF YOU DO NOT HAVE ANY TAMARIND USE LEMON OR LIME JUICE INSTEAD.

SERVES 4

250g/9oz firm tofu dried and cut into 2cm/¾ in cubes
2 tbsp olive oil
100g/3½oz chestnut or shitake mushrooms sliced
2 tbsp chopped coriander
100g/3½oz watercress, large stems removed
1 red chilli finely sliced
For the stock:
2 tbsp tamarind pulp
2 dried red chillies
2 kafir lime leaves OR 2 tsp grated lime zest
2 tbsp grated ginger
1 onion cut into quarters
1Lt/1¾ pt/35 fl oz water

Put all of the ingredients for the stock into a saucepan and bring them to the boil. Reduce the heat and simmer for 10 minutes.

While the stock is cooking heat 1 tbsp oil oil in a frying pan and sauté the mushrooms over a medium heat for 5 minutes. Remove and put to one side.

Add the rest of the oil to the frying pan and fry the tofu over a medium heat for 5 minutes turning it over to seal it on all sides.

Strain the stock and return it to the saucepan. Add the mushrooms and the watercress and bring the soup back to the boil. Stir in the sliced chilli and tofu and turn off the heat. Serve garnished with the chopped coriander.

Whole grains, seeds & cereals

Oatmeal, Quinoa, Millet, Buckwheat, Bulgar Wheat, Pearl Spelt, Pearl Barley and Amaranth

Why?

It is thought that early man consumed between 50 and 100 grams of starchy carbohydrate a day. This carbohydrate would have been complex and unrefined. It would have been obtained from a wide range of different grains, cereals, seeds and tubers. Today on average people who eat a typical western diet are consuming between 350 and 600 grams of carbohydrates a day and almost all of this is in a highly refined form that our body quickly converts into sugar. This is a massive increase that we are just not designed to cope with, so it is hardly surprising that many of us are either insulin resistant or close to becoming insulin resistant.

We all need carbohydrates in our diet so eating sensible amounts of carbohydrates is fine, provided they are unrefined. Because unrefined carbohydrates take longer to break down and digest than refined carbohydrates they release their glucose slowly. This results in insulin being better regulated as it is released slowly in line with the release of the glucose. Because complex carbohydrates are essentially the complete seed of a plant, they contain a surprising amount of protein, vitamins, minerals and fibre and the fibre means that when you eat complex carbohydrates you feel full for much longer.

As with so many other things not all whole grains are created equal. Some are much better than others in terms of the amount of protein they contain and some are better than others in terms of fibre, minerals and trace elements. Without exception they all contain far more nutrients than refined grains and polished rice. As a general rule these complex carbohydrates contain between 100kcal and 1550kcal per 100 gram when cooked. Their protein content varies but it is worth noting that the protein they do contain is very easy to digest.

Once upon a time whole grains and cereals were our staple food. Sadly now, for many if not most of us, they no longer have a place on our menus

Oats in the form of oatmeal

For some people oatmeal is a 'superfood'. It is high in fibre, low in fat and high in protein. One hundred grams of uncooked oatmeal contains 11 grams of protein and just under 10 grams of fibre.

Why do some people regard oatmeal as a superfood? There are quite a few reasons.

- Oatmeal contains high levels of magnesium and as magnesium is needed for the production of insulin, it is thought that foods high in magnesium help stabilise blood sugar and reduce the risk of type 2 diabetes developing.
- Many studies have shown that a fibre called beta-glucan, that is unique to oatmeal, has a beneficial effect on cholesterol levels. It also contains an antioxidant called avenanthramide that again is unique to oatmeal, and this prevents free radicals from oxidising and damaging cholesterol.
- Oatmeal contains compounds called plant lignans which are converted in our digestive tract into mammalian lignans. One of these is called enterolactone and it is thought that this is able to protect us against heart disease and some cancers.

The larger the 'flake' the less processed the oatmeal is, the more nutrients it retains and the slower it is to digest. You can make your own muesli or granola by adding nuts and dried fruit to raw or toasted oatmeal, and good old fashioned porridge, made with milk or water, is a healthy start to the day that has stood the test of time. You can use oatmeal to make muesli bars and flapjacks and 'pin head' oatmeal makes wonderful oatcakes.

Toasting Oatmeal

Having a supply of oatmeal that is already toasted is well worthwhile as it is a useful store cupboard ingredient. It is a good alternative to breadcrumbs for making toppings for gratins and it works really well when mixed with pesto as a topping. It can also be used in biscuits and desserts.

You can either grill the oatmeal or toast it in a dry pan on the hob.

To grill the oatmeal pre heat the grill on high and put the oatmeal in a thin layer on a tray. Grill under a high heat for 3 to 4 minutes, stirring it and turning it over every minute. Keep you eye on it as it burns very easily. When it is ready it should be a light golden brown.

To toast the oatmeal on the hob pre heat a pan over a medium heat and when it is hot put in the oatmeal. Keep stirring it around. It should take about 5 minutes to turn golden brown. Once it has cooled down you will need to store the oatmeal in an airtight container.

Quinoa

Quinoa, pronounced "keen-wah" has been eaten for 5,000 years by the people of South America. It is not a grain but a seed from a vegetable that is closely related to Swiss Chard. Like other whole grains quinoa is high in protein. One hundred grams of uncooked quinoa contains 14 grams of protein and this is close to the protein content of milk. The protein in quinoa is also a complete protein as it contains all of the essential amino acids. Quinoa is gluten free and a good source of calcium.

One thing to remember about quinoa is that it is coated with an anti-nutrient called saponin. Even though the quinoa you buy will have been washed it is important that you wash it well before cooking it. Rinse the grain in at least two changes of water.

Cooking Quinoa

Quinoa is not the easiest of grains to cook as it needs long, very slow cooking. The best way to cook it is by using the absorption method. One part quinoa needs just slightly under two parts of water. The easiest way to do this is to use a small 5fl oz/150 ml dish like a ramekin dish. This holds about 100g/3½ oz of quinoa.

You can cook quinoa on the hob or in the microwave.

To cook it on the hob, put the quinoa into a saucepan, bring it to the boil, cover with a tight fitting lid and reduce to a very low heat. Leave it to cook for 20 – 25 minutes. When it has finished cooking leave it to stand for at least a quarter of an hour before taking off the lid.

To cook it in the microwave, put the quinoa into a microwave bowl with the water. Cover it loosely and microwave on full power for 10 minutes. Give it a stir, put the cover back on and leave it to stand for 10 minutes. Then microwave it again on full power for 4 minutes and leave it to stand for 5 minutes before serving.

Troublesome it may be to cook, but cooked quinoa freezes well. To freeze quinoa all you need to do is open freeze it on a large tray lined with cling film or non stick foil and when it is frozen put it into a box or a bag so that you can use it as and when needed. It thaws out very quickly once it is taken out of the freezer.

Millet

Millet is a gluten free wholegrain that has a sweet nutty flavour. Like Quinoa it is high in protein. As 100 gram of uncooked millet contains around 11% protein it makes a valuable addition to your diet. Like oatmeal it contains antioxidants and high levels of magnesium. Millet is the staple food of millions of people around the world and like quinoa and oatmeal it is a grain that has stood the test of time. You can use millet in exactly the same way as you would use rice and other grains, hot or cold in salads.

Like most grains the best way to cook millet is by using the absorption method. Like quinoa one part millet needs about two parts of water. The easiest way to do this is to use a small 5fl oz/150 ml ramekin dish. This holds about 100g/3½ oz of millet.

Cooking Millet

To cook it on the hob, put the millet into a saucepan, bring it to the boil, cover with a tight fitting lid and turn off the heat. Leave the millet to soak for 10 minutes. Bring it back to the boil and reduce the heat to very low. Leave the millet to cook for 20 to 25 minutes. When it has finished cooking add a tablespoon of boiling water, put the lid back on and leave it to stand for a quarter of an hour before taking off the lid. Like quinoa millet freezes well so it is worth cooking it in a large batch and then freezing it in small portions.

Pearl Spelt

Spelt is one of the oldest cultivated crops that is thought to go back back between 7,000 and 8,000 years. It was an important staple food in parts of Europe from the Bronze Age through to the Middle Ages. Spelt is closely related to the 'bread wheat' we know today. It survived as a relic crop and has now been revived as a healthy alternative to wheat because of the amount of protein and fibre it contains. One hundred grams of uncooked pearl spelt contains 14½ grams of protein and 10 grams of fibre. You can use it instead of rice, it makes excellent risottos and once cooked it freezes well.

Pearl Barley

Pearl barley is barley that has been hulled, rolled to remove the bran and then polished.

It is the most common form of barley to be eaten because it cooks quickly and is less chewy than barley that has only had the hull removed. As well as being used in soups, stews and casseroles, pearl barley can be used to make risottos. The classic Italian dish orzotto is made from barley. Like pearl spelt pearl barley freezes well and can be used instead of rice.

Cooking Pearl Barley & Pearl Spelt

These are best covered with cold water, brought to the boil and then simmered slowly. Make sure you wash the spelt or barley well before cooking it as it tends to be quite dusty. Pearl Spelt needs to simmer for about 20 minutes but pearl barley will need to simmer for between 45 and 50 minutes before it is cooked.

Buckwheat in the form of buckwheat 'groats'

Despite its name buckwheat is not a grain and it is not related to wheat. It is the seed of a plant that is related to sorrel, knot weed and rhubarb. Buckwheat is thought to have first been cultivated in south east Asia around 6,000 years ago. From there it spread to Central Asia, the Middle East and Europe. It was one of the first crops brought to America by the European settlers. While its cultivation declined in the west in the 20th century it remained a staple food in Russia and northern European countries. One hundred grams of uncooked buckwheat contains 13 grams of protein and 10 grams of fibre.

Cooking Whole Buckwheat

Unlike millet and quinoa whole buckwheat is best covered with cold water, brought to the boil and then simmered very gently for between 20 to 25 minutes. Drain before serving.

Amaranth

Amaranth is another ancient grain that goes back around 8,000 years. It was cultivated by the Aztecs and the people of Mexico and Central America. It is also grown in northern India. Over the years cultivation declined in favour of corn and wheat but with increased demand for healthier food cultivation began again in the early 1970's. Amaranth has a nutty earthy flavour. One hundred grams of uncooked amaranth contains 13½ grams of protein and like quinoa the protein is a complete protein.

Bulgar wheat

Bulgar wheat is widely used in the Middle East, Eastern Europe and Indian cooking. It is made from different varieties of locally grown wheat. The wheat is hulled and either left whole or cracked. It is available as fine, medium or coarse. It is quick and easy to cook and this makes it a convenient and versatile food. One hundred grams of uncooked bulgar wheat contains 12 grams of protein and 18 grams of fibre.

Cooking Bulgar Wheat

For all types of bulgar wheat add 1 part bulgar wheat to 2 parts water. A small ramekin dish is about 100 grams of bulgar wheat. For fine bulgar wheat bring the water to the boil, add the bulgar wheat, give it a stir, cover it and leave it to stand for 5 – 10 minutes. Medium bulgar wheat needs to be brought to the boil and then gently simmered for 5 minutes before being left to stand. Course bulgar wheat needs to be brought to the boil and then simmered for 10 minutes.

Couscous.

Couscous is not a whole grain but as it is quick and easy to prepare it is a useful store cupboard ingredient. Couscous is made from wheat and sometimes barley. It comes in fine, medium and giant forms. Because it it pre-processed couscous is by far the easiest 'grain' to prepare. Like bulgar wheat all you need to do is add 1 part couscous to 2 parts boiling water, give it a stir and then leave it to stand for 5 – 10 minutes. Medium couscous needs to be gently simmered for 5 minutes before being left to stand. Giant couscous needs to be simmered for 10 minutes.

Mixed Grains

Because all grains freeze well it is well worth preparing a supply of mixed grains and keeping them in the freezer. Mix together different combinations of cooked quinoa, barley, buckwheat and bulgar wheat and put them into bags in portions that meet your need. All grains can be used from frozen or thawed out in the microwave when needed.

Toasted Oatmeal Coating

THIS IS A USEFUL MIXTURE OF OATMEAL, SPICES AND SEEDS THAT CAN BE USED AS A CRUNCHY TOPPING FOR BAKES AND GRATINS AND AS A COATING FOR BURGERS.

SERVES 4
200g/7oz flaked oatmeal
3 tbsp olive oil
3 tbsp water
A handful of sunflower seeds
½ tsp ground turmeric
1 tsp garlic granules
1 tbsp dried oregano
1 tsp chilli flakes

Pre heat the oven to 160°C/ 325°F/Gas 3

Grease a 20cm/8 in square baking tin and line the base with baking parchment or non stick foil.

Mix the flaked oats and sunflower seeds with the turmeric, garlic granules, chilli flakes and oregano.

Put the water and olive oil into a saucepan and bring it to the boil.

Add the oil and water to the flaked oats. Mix well and press the mixture into the prepared tin. Bake for 30 minutes until the oats are golden brown.

Leave the oats to cool completely, then use a rolling pin to break the oats down into large crumbs. Store in an airtight tin or in the freezer.

Quinoa, Avocado, Feta & Tomato Salad

YOU CAN USE FRESH BABY PLUM TOMATOES OR SUN DRIED TOMATOES TO MAKE THIS. THE SUN DRIED TOMATOES GIVE THE SALAD A MORE INTENSE FLAVOUR.

SERVES 4
100g/3½oz quinoa
Just under 300ml/10 fl oz water
3 large ripe avocados
200g/7oz feta cut into 5mm/¼ in dice
400g/14oz can red beans drained and rinsed
Small bunch chives finely sliced
200g/7 oz baby plum tomatoes OR some sun dried tomatoes cut into quarters
30g/1oz rocket or watercress
2 tbsp lemon or lime juice

Wash the quinoa and drain it. Put it into a saucepan, bring it to the boil, cover with a tight fitting lid and reduce to a very low heat. Leave it to cook for 25 – 30 minutes. When it has finished cooking leave it to stand for at least half an hour before taking off the lid.

Alternatively microwave the quinoa following the instructions at the beginning of this section.

Cut the avocados in half, remove the stone using a small spoon then peel the avocados, cut them into 1 cm/½ in dice and cover them with the lemon or lime juice.

When the quinoa is cold mix everything together in a large bowl.

Classic Soda Bread

TRADITIONALLY SODA BREAD IS MADE WITH BUTTERMILK. AS BUTTERMILK IS DIFFICULT TO FIND THESE DAYS, USE A MIXTURE OF NATURAL UNSWEETENED YOGHURT AND WATER INSTEAD. SODA BREAD MADE FROM WHOLEGRAIN WHEAT OR SPELT NEVER RISES AS WELL AS SODA BREAD MADE WITH WHITE FLOUR BUT IT TASTES MUCH BETTER AND IT MAKES WONDERFUL TOAST.

ANY BREAD MADE WITH CHEMICAL RAISING AGENTS NEEDS TO GO INTO A VERY HOT OVEN AS SOON AS THE DOUGH IS MIXED. IT SHOULD ONLY BE KNEADED LIGHTLY, JUST LONG ENOUGH TO SHAPE IT. THIS IS BECAUSE THE RAISING AGENT STARTS WORKING AS SOON AS IT COMES INTO CONTACT WITH FLUID, SO EXTENDED KNEADING MEANS THAT YOU END UP WITH A LOAF THAT DOES NOT RISE WELL.

500g/1lb 2oz wholegrain spelt
2 tsp bicarbonate of soda
Hand full of pumpkin seeds
Hand full sunflower seeds
200ml/7 fl oz natural unsweetened yoghurt
200ml/7 fl oz water

You will need a lightly greased baking tray and a 24cm/10in cake tin with a solid base to make this. Putting the cake tin upside down on top of the bread will help it rise.

Pre heat the oven to 220°C/ 450°F/Gas 6.

Mix together the spelt, bicarbonate of soda and seeds in a large bowl.

Whisk the yoghurt and water together and add this to the flour. Mix it well, turn it onto a floured board and quickly shape it into a round.

Put the dough onto the baking tray, cover it with the inverted cake tin and put it into the oven. Bake for 30 minutes. Remove the tin and reduce the temperature to 180°C/ 350°F/Gas 4. Cook for another 10 – 15 minutes.

When it is cooked the bread should sound hollow when the base is tapped.

Date & Muesli Bars

THESE ARE MOIST CHEWY BISCUITS THAT ARE QUICK AND EASY TO MAKE AND THEY KEEP FOR UP TO A WEEK IN AN AIRTIGHT TIN. THE MASHED BANANA WORKS WONDERS AS IT TAKES THE PLACE OF EGG AND BINDS THE INGREDIENTS TOGETHER.

Makes 9 - 16
2 large ripe bananas
1 heaped tbsp dark unrefined Muscavado sugar
2 tbsp olive oil
120g/4¼ oz chopped dates
30g/1oz pumpkin seeds
3 tsp mixed spice
½ tsp ground ginger
200g/7oz flaked oatmeal
50g/1¾oz chopped pecan nuts or walnuts

You will need a 20cm/8 in greased square tin, preferably silicon bakeware.

Pre heat the oven to 160°C/ 325°F/Gas 3.

Put the bananas into a bowl and use a hand blender to whiz them into a smooth purée. Add the olive oil and blend until well mixed.

Mix together the flaked oatmeal, muscavado sugar, mixed spice and ground ginger in a separate bowl. If the sugar is lumpy break it up with your fingers.

Stir in the nuts, pumpkin seeds and chopped dates.

Add the banana and oil to the oatmeal, seeds and nuts and mix thoroughly. The mixture will be fairly dry. Put it into the prepared tin and, using the back of a spoon, press it down firmly.

Cook for 30 minutes until the biscuit is firm to the touch and beginning to look slightly golden around the edge. Take it out of the oven and put to one side to cool a little.

When it is cool enough to handle put the biscuit onto a chopping board and use a sharp knife to cut it into 9 or16 pieces.

Kedgeree

KEDGEREE IS TRADITIONALLY MADE FROM BASMATI RICE AND SMOKED HADDOCK. THIS RECIPE IS MADE FROM BUCKWHEAT AND SMOKED MACKEREL. THE KEDGEREE WILL TASTE JUST AS GOOD IF IT IS MADE WITH SALMON, TROUT OR SMOKED HADDOCK. INSTEAD OF BUCKWHEAT YOU CAN USE PEARL SPELT, RICE, PEARL BARLEY OR QUINOA. THE NUTTY TASTE OF BUCKWHEAT WORKS REALLY WELL WITH THE SMOKED MACKEREL.

SERVES 4

200g/7oz buckwheat
1 tsp turmeric
3 bay leaves
200g/7oz hot smoked mackerel
4 hard boiled eggs, peeled and cut into quarters
1 large white onion finely sliced
1 large stick of celery chopped
Juice of a lemon
2 tbsp olive oil
1 tsp ground cardamom
2 tbsp chopped dill
1 tbsp chopped parsley
100g/3½oz frozen peas
200g/7oz mange tout cut in half lengthways

You will need a large frying pan or a chefs pan with a lid to make this.

Put the buckwheat into a saucepan, add the turmeric and bay leaves, cover it with plenty of water and bring it to the boil. When the buckwheat is boiling reduce the heat, cover it and simmer it for 20 minutes. Drain, remove the bay leaves and put the buckwheat to one side.

Take the skin off of the smoked mackerel and break up the fillets into bite size pieces.

Heat the oil in a frying pan and sauté the onion and celery on a medium heat for 5 minutes until they are tender.

Add the ground cardamom and stir in the cooked buckwheat. Add 2 tbsp water and lay the pieces of mackerel on top. Put the lid on a leave the buckwheat and fish to heat through over a low heat for a few minutes while you cook the peas and mange tout.

Put the peas into a microwave bowl with 2 tbsp water, cover and microwave on full power for 4 minutes. Add the mange tout, replace the cover and cook for another minute.

Strain the peas and mange tout and stir them into the mackerel and buckwheat. Turn off the heat, arrange the hard boiled eggs on top and scatter over the chopped dill and parsley.

Courgette Crown Bread

ADDING GRATED COURGETTE AND CHEESE CAN TRANSFORM AN ORDINARY LOAF INTO SOMETHING SPECIAL. USE YELLOW COURGETTES IF YOU CAN GET THEM.

450g/1 lb grated courgette
500g/1lb 2oz whole grain spelt
Sachet fast acting bakers yeast
4 tbsp finely grated parmesan
1 tbsp sesame seeds
½ tsp cayenne pepper
1 tsp garlic granules (optional)
2 tbsp olive oil
Tepid water

You will need a 23cm/9 in round tin to make this. If you are using a metal tin grease it well.

Mix the spelt with the yeast, cayenne pepper, parmesan and garlic granules if you are using them.

Add the grated courgette and mix it into the flour.

Slowly add some tepid water and mix the dough with your hands until you have a firm dough. How much water you need depends on the amount of fluid in the courgettes.

Knead the dough on a floured board for about 10 minutes until it is smooth and 'stretchy'. Cover and leave the dough to prove until it has doubled in size.

Knead the dough for a couple of minutes and divide it into 8 pieces and roll these into balls. Put one ball in the centre of the baking tin and arrange the others around the outside. Brush with milk or water and sprinkle the sesame seeds over the top. Cover and leave the bread to rise until it has doubled in size.

Pre heat the oven to 200°C/ 400°F/Gas 5 and bake the bread for 30 minutes. It is cooked when it sounds hollow when you tap the bottom.

Mushroom, Buckwheat & Walnut Roast

THIS IS A RICH DARK BAKE THAT CAN BE SERVED EITHER HOT OR COLD. THE MAIN INGREDIENTS ARE BUCKWHEAT, PECAN NUTS, WALNUTS, MUSHROOMS AND SPINACH. YOU CAN USE FRESH SPINACH BUT IN ORDER TO MAKE IT QUICK AND SIMPLE THIS RECIPE USES FROZEN SPINACH.

SERVES 4

110g/4oz buckwheat
110g/4oz white onions finely chopped
225g/8oz chestnut mushrooms
110g/4oz walnuts or pecan nuts
8oz frozen leaf spinach
1 tsp dried rosemary
1 tsp dried sage
1 large free range egg
1 tbsp butter or ghee
salt and ground black pepper to taste

Grease a 900g/2lb loaf tin and pre heat the oven to 180°C/ 350°F/Gas 4.

Wash the buckwheat in several changes of water. Drain, put it into a saucepan and cover it with water. Bring it to the boil, cover and simmer for 20 minutes. Drain and put to one side.

Cook the frozen spinach following the instructions on the packet. Put it into a sieve and drain really well.

Heat the butter in a saucepan and sauté the chopped onions for 2 -3 minutes, then add the sliced mushrooms, the rosemary and the sage. Give everything a good stir, put on the lid, turn down the heat and cook for 10 minutes.

Grind the walnuts or pecan nuts. Beat the egg. Mix the mushroom and onions with the cooked buckwheat, add the spinach, ground nuts and mix with the beaten egg.

Press the mixture into the loaf tin and bake for 50 to 60 minutes. Leave to rest for 10 minutes before removing it from the tin.

Tabbouleh with Borlotti Bean Paté

TABBOULEH IS TRADITIONALLY MADE WITH BULGAR WHEAT BUT YOU CAN ALSO USE QUINOA OR COUSCOUS. THIS RECIPE USES COARSE BULGAR WHEAT AND THIS NEEDS COOKING. IF YOU USE FINE OR MEDIUM BULGAR WHEAT ALL YOU NEED TO DO IS SOAK IT IN BOILING WATER FOR 10 MINUTES. SERVE THE TABBOULEH ON ITS OWN, WITH BORLOTTI BEAN PATE OR WITH MISO, TOFU & TAHINI DIP.

SERVES 4
FOR THE TABBOULEH
200g/7oz coarse bulgar wheat

400ml/14fl oz water

1 tsp vegetable stock powder

500g/1lb 2oz chopped ripe vine tomatoes

Small bunch flat leaf parsley finely chopped

55g/2oz fresh coriander or mint finely chopped

1 telegraph cucumber peeled, de-seeded and finely chopped

4 tbsp olive oil

2 tbsp capers

Juice of a lemon

Salt and pepper to taste

FOR THE BORLOTTI BEAN PATE
400g 14oz can of Borlotti beans

3 tbsp natural unsweetened yoghurt OR soft cheese like ricotta

Juice of a lemon

½ tsp chilli paste, Sambol Oelek or some finely chopped red chilli

1 clove crushed garlic

10 sun dried tomatoes

12 stoned salted black olives

8 basil leaves

To make the Tabbouleh.

Bring the water and vegetable stock powder to the boil. Add the bulgar wheat and bring it back to the boil. Turn the heat to low, cover and leave it to cook very gently for 10 minutes. Turn off the heat and leave it to stand covered for at least 15 minutes before removing the lid.

When the bulgar wheat is cool stir in the tomatoes, cucumber, parsley, mint and olive oil, lemon juice and season to taste. You can store the Tabbouleh in the fridge for up to 2 days.

To make the Borlotti bean paté.

Drain and rinse the Borlotti beans and place them with the lemon juice, yoghurt or soft cheese, chilli and crushed garlic in a deep bowl. Whiz them with a blender until they are a smooth purée.

Chop the sun dried tomatoes and black olives and shred the basil leaves. Mix the olives, basil and tomatoes with the bean purée. Cover and chill until needed.

Sometimes Eat

Rice

Why?

Rice is the staple food of millions of people around the world and it is cheap and easy to cook. However, it contains large amounts of glycemic starch, a starch that is a converted into sugar and absorbed almost as quickly as the sugar in a soft drink. One hundred grams of uncooked white rice contains about 80 grams of carbohydrate, around 7 grams of protein and only 1.3 grams of dietary fibre and it is the small amount of fibre that is the problem with white rice. As most of the fibre, vitamins and minerals in rice are in the layer of husk and bran that is removed when the rice is polished, it is not surprising that brown rice is far more nutritious than white rice. Interestingly, because some of the oils in the husk and bran oxidise, brown rice has a much shorter shelf life than polished white rice.

Eating boiled rice as a staple food is something of a paradox. We are told to be careful about how much rice we eat as it 'makes us fat' and yet Asians, Chinese and Japanese eat it two or three times a day and as a general rule they stay slim. How and why this happens is unclear but what is clear is that scientists have now discovered a way of improving the nutritional content of rice by cooking it in a different way. Simply by adding a small amount of butter, olive oil or coconut oil to the water the rice is cooked in and then cooking the rice, cooling it quickly and leaving it in the fridge for 12 to 24 hours, some of the glycemic starch in the rice is changed into resistant starch, a fibre that we digest slowly. As well as slowing down the rate at which the glucose is released from the rice, this fibre also acts as a prebiotic fibre that supports the growth of healthy bacteria in your digestive tract. Contrary to what you would expect, reheating the rice when you are ready to eat it increases the amount of resistant starch even more.

Should you worry about the arsenic in rice?

As well as being toxic arsenic is also a major carcinogen. Just about all soil and water contains arsenic and small amounts find their way into our food. Usually there is not enough arsenic to worry about but because rice is grown in water it contains between ten and twenty times more arsenic than other cereals. The World Health Organisation and the EU have both set guidelines for the amount of arsenic that is permitted, both in rice itself and products like rice cakes and rice milk that are made from rice. However there is some debate about whether the permitted levels of arsenic are actually safe.

As with vitamins, minerals and fibre the husk and bran of rice contains a lot of the arsenic so brown rice contains more than white rice. For most of us if we eat rice in moderation as part of a balanced diet the amount of arsenic we consume should not be a problem. There is however, something you can do about it and, as with fibre, it is all to do with the way the rice is cooked. Even if you rinse it first, cooking rice by the absorption method means that all of the arsenic stays in the rice. If you boil the rice in plenty of water and then rinse it about half of the arsenic is removed. However, if you soak the rice overnight and then rinse it before boiling it in plenty of water between 70% and 80% of the arsenic will be removed. So if you add some fat or oil to the cooking water and then rinse the rice in cold water before keeping it in the fridge, you remove most of the arsenic, increase the amount of resistant starch the rice contains and transform it into a much healthier food.

How

Instead of being quick and easy to cook soaking, boiling and rinsing makes cooking rice a bit of a chore, but provided the rice is cooled quickly cooked rice can be safely kept for up to two days in a covered container in the fridge. But the good news is that rice freezes really well and you can use it straight from the freezer.

Broccoli Risotto Torte

THIS IS A SAVOURY 'CAKE' THAT IS SERVED CUT INTO WEDGES. IT CAN BE EATEN HOT OR COLD AND NEEDS ONLY A SALAD AS AN ACCOMPANIMENT. YOU CAN MAKE THE TORTE WITH BARLEY, SPELT, BUCKWHEAT, QUINOA OR RISOTTO RICE. THE CAKE HAS A SOFTER TEXTURE WHEN IT IS MADE WITH RICE. THIS IS A GOOD WAY TO 'STRETCH OUT' THE RICE AS THE RISOTTO CAKE WILL EASILY SERVE 8 PEOPLE OR MORE.

SERVES 8

225g/8oz risotto rice
1 tbsp olive oil
1 large onion peeled and finely chopped
50g/1½oz butter
1 tsp cayenne pepper
450g/1lb broccoli broken into florets
1 large courgette quartered length ways and chopped into 1cm/½ in chunks
100g/3½oz grated parmesan or pecorino
4 large free range eggs separated

Cook the rice in plenty of water and a tablespoon of olive oil. Cooking times vary but most risotto rice will be cooked in about 15 minutes. Rinse the rice twice in cold water and drain it well. You can cook the rice a day before and leave it overnight in the fridge.

Grease a 25cm/10in round deep cake tin, a silicon baking tin is ideal.

Pre heat the oven to 180°C/ 350°F/Gas 4.

Melt the butter in a small saucepan, add the onion and sauté it on a medium heat for 5 minutes, then add the cayenne pepper

Blanch the broccoli in boiling water for 3 minutes. Drain and refresh in cold water.

Put the courgette into a microwave bowl, cover and cook on full power for 3 minutes.

Whisk the egg whites in a clean, dry bowl until they are stiff and form soft peaks.

Add the egg yolks and grated cheese to the rice and mix well. Then stir in the cooked onions, the broccoli and then courgettes.

Add a third of the whisked egg whites and stir until everything is thoroughly mixed. Now gently fold in the remaining egg whites.

Pour the mixture into the cake tin, cover with foil and bake for 45 minutes. Take off the foil, put back into the oven and cook for another 15 minutes.

Broad Bean & Almond Pilaf

THIS CAN BE COOKED IN ADVANCE AND REHEATED WHEN YOU ARE READY TO SERVE IT. YOU CAN USE QUINOA, BASMATI RICE, PEARL BARLEY, SPELT OR BUCKWHEAT TO MAKE THIS.

SERVES 4

200g/7oz basmati rice
1 tbsp olive oil
300g/10½oz frozen broad beans
2 tbsp olive oil
3 medium white onions finely sliced
3 cloves garlic crushed
1 tsp vegetable stock powder
1 tsp cayenne pepper
1 tbsp cumin seeds
3 tbsp raisins
40g/1½ oz flaked almonds
2 tbsp lemon juice
Salt and pepper to taste

Cook the rice in plenty of water and a tablespoon of olive oil. Cooking times vary but most basmati rice will be cooked in about 10 minutes. Rinse the rice twice in cold water and drain it well. You can cook the rice a day before and leave it overnight in the fridge.

Pre heat the oven to 180°C/ 350°F/Gas 4

Put the almonds onto a baking try and cook them for 7 to 8 minutes until they are light golden brown.

Sauté the onions in the oil over a medium heat for 5 minutes. Add the garlic, cayenne pepper and cumin seeds and cook for 2 – 3 minutes.

Stir in the rice and the raisins. Turn off the heat and leave the lid on the pan while you cook the broad beans.

Bring the broad beans to the boil and cook for 6 - 7 minutes. Drain them and, if you are an advocate of peeled broad beans you can peel them. Add the broad beans to the rice and raisins, then tip everything into a micro wave serving dish. Cover and microwave on full power for 3 minutes. Stir in the lemon juice. Sprinkle the toasted almonds on top and serve.

Pasta – in any shape you want

Why?

Pasta comes in many different shapes and sizes and in different colours and flavours. Whole wheat pasta contains more vitamins and minerals than white pasta and between two and three times more fibre. Even though white pasta is made from refined wheat, it takes longer to digest and release its sugar than other refined carbohydrates. This appears to be because of the stretching and rolling process the pasta goes through when it is made. This entraps some of the starch granules in a sponge like network of protein molecules in the pasta dough. Asian noodles such as udon and rice vermicelli also share the same characteristic.

Pasta is quick and easy to prepare. It should always be cooked al dente or 'firm to bite', in other words it should be slightly firm and offer some resistance when you chew it. This is the best way to eat it as the more it is cooked the easier and quicker it is to digest. As well as eating it 'al dente' there is something else you can do to improve the nutritional content of pasta. As with rice, cooking the pasta and then leaving it to cool transforms some of the glycemic starch into resistant starch. So simply by cooking pasta, rinsing it in cold water, popping it into the fridge for a few hours and then reheating it when you are ready to eat it makes it a much healthier food.

How:

Although most manufacturers specify a cooking time, when you cook pasta start testing it 2 to 3 minutes before the recommended time is up. The only thing to be mindful of is the total amount of pasta you eat. Pasta is high in carbohydrates and low in nutrients, so go for more vegetables and less pasta.

Salmon Pasta & Red Pepper Sauce

IDEALLY THE RED PEPPERS SHOULD BE ROASTED AND THEN PEELED BEFORE BEING BLENDED INTO THE YOGHURT. HOWEVER, THE RECIPE WORKS JUST AS WELL IF THE PEPPERS ARE SAUTÉED WITH HALF A TEASPOON OF SMOKED PAPRIKA. YOU CAN USE ANY TYPE OF LARGE, CHUNKY PASTA, COOK IT IN ADVANCE AND HEAT IT THROUGH WHEN YOU ARE READY TO SERVE.

SERVES 4

700g/1 lb 9oz salmon
3 large red peppers
3 tbsp olive oil
1 medium white or red onion roughly chopped
1 clove garlic crushed (optional)
1 tsp Sambol Oelek or chilli paste
90ml/3 fl oz dry white wine or water
½ tsp smoked paprika
125ml/4 fl oz natural unsweetened Greek style yoghurt
Salt and pepper to taste
200g/7oz Rigatoni
70g/2½oz baby spinach
Finely chopped parsley or chervil to garnish

Skin and bone the salmon and cut it into 2cm/¾ in pieces.

Cut the peppers in half, de-seed them and slice them thinly.

Heat 1 tbsp of the olive oil in a saucepan on a fairly high heat and add the peppers. Stir fry for 5 minutes to bring out the flavour of the peppers but don't let them brown.

Take out half of the peppers and put them to one side. Add the chopped onion and add the crushed garlic. Turn down the heat, stir for a minute and then add the white wine or water. Bring to the boil, cover, reduce the heat and simmer for 15 minutes. Turn off the heat and leave the peppers in the saucepan.

Cook the pasta in line with the instructions on the packet. Just make sure it is 'al dente' and still has some bite when you have finished cooking it. Stir in the baby spinach and leave the spinach to wilt for a minute before you drain the pasta. Stir the reserved peppers and a tablespoon of olive oil into the drained pasta to prevent it sticking together.

While the pasta is cooking, heat the remaining oil over a medium heat in a non stick frying pan. Add the salmon and cook for 5 minutes until it is just set.

Add the yoghurt to the peppers in the saucepan and use a hand blender to blend the peppers into a thick sauce. Mix a quarter of this into the pasta, spinach and peppers.

Add the cooked salmon to the rest of the pepper sauce and gently stir it in. Serve the pasta and wilted spinach with the salmon and red pepper sauce on top.

A Hearty Italian Hotpot

THIS IS AN ADAPTATION OF A CLASSIC ITALIAN VEGETABLE STEW CALLED 'PASTA A FAGLIO'. THE AUTHENTIC DISH USES DRIED BORLOTTI BEANS BUT CHICKPEAS ALSO WORK WELL. CANNED BEANS ARE MUCH QUICKER THAN PREPARING DRIED BEANS WHICH NEED SOAKING OVERNIGHT BEFORE THEY ARE COOKED. YOU CAN COOK THE PASTA IN ADVANCE AND ADD IT TO THE HOTPOT AT THE LAST MINUTE.

SERVES 6

2 x 400g/14 ox can of borlotti beans or chickpeas drained and rinsed
1 large onion finely sliced
3 tbsp olive oil
1 large leek finely sliced
2 large carrots peeled and finely chopped
2 sticks celery finely chopped
1 large potato peeled and chopped into 1cm/½ in dice
4 cloves of garlic crushed
1Lt/1¾ pt/35 fl oz vegetable stock
½ tsp dried thyme
½ tsp dried rosemary
½ tsp dried sage
200g/7oz conchiglie or small pasta shells
10 large tomatoes each cut into 8 pieces
2 tbsp tomato purée
Salt and ground black pepper
Finely grated parmesan and finely
Chopped parsley or chervil to serve

Heat the olive oil in a large saucepan and add the sliced onions, leeks, potatoes and carrots. Sauté for 5 minutes and then add the garlic, thyme, rosemary and sage.

Stir in the vegetable stock, the tomato purée and the borlotti beans. Bring to the boil, reduce the heat, cover and leave the 'stew' simmering while you cook the pasta.

Add the pasta to a large saucepan of boiling water. Cook for 7 to 8 minutes until it is just cooked, then drain it.

Add the pasta to the bean stew and stir in the tomatoes. Scatter some chopped parsley and grated parmesan over the top and serve the rest of the parmesan in a separate bowl.

Courgette & Red Pepper Lasagne

READY TO USE LASAGNE MAKES LASAGNE FAIRLY QUICK AND EASY TO MAKE. EVEN THOUGH THE INSTRUCTIONS ON THE PACKET DO NOT TELL YOU TO, PRE-SOAKING THE SHEETS OF LASAGNE WHILE YOU PREPARE THE FILLING IMPROVES THE TEXTURE. YOU WILL NEED A 5CM/2 IN DEEP LARGE OVENPROOF DISH OR CASSEROLE THAT TAKES 3 SHEETS OF LASAGNE ACROSS THE BASE TO MAKE THIS. A DISH THAT IS 24CM X 20 CM OR 10 IN X 8 IN IS IDEAL. YOU WILL FIND THE RECIPE FOR BASIL PESTO IN THE HERBS AND SPICES SECTION.

SERVES 6

9 sheets ready to use lasagne
6 spring onions finely sliced
1 clove garlic crushed (optional)
400g/14 oz can chopped tomatoes
3 tbsp tomato purée
1 tsp cayenne pepper
4 tbsp fromage frais or natural unsweetened yoghurt
3 large free range eggs
3 tbsp finely grated parmesan.
2 large red peppers
400g/14 oz courgettes thinly sliced
For the topping:
350g/12oz packet silken tofu
100ml/3½ fl oz milk
1 large free range egg
60g/2¼oz basil pesto
3 tbsp finely grated parmesan

Pre heat the oven to 200°C/ 400°F/Gas 5 and grease the baking dish.

Put the sheets of lasagne into a large shallow bowl and cover them with hot water. Leave them to soak while you prepare the filling.

Cut the red peppers into quarters and remove the seeds. Put them onto a baking tray lined with non stick foil and roast them for 20 to 25 minutes. Tip them into a bowl and cover them with cling film.

Put the sliced courgette into a microwave bowl, cover and cook for 3 minutes until it is just beginning to soften.

Whisk the eggs, tomato purée, cayenne pepper, fromage frais and parmesan together. Stir in the spring onions, the copped tomatoes and the garlic. If there is any fluid in the bowl with the courgettes drain this off and stir this in as well.

When the peppers are cool enough to handle remove the cling film and peel off the skin. You do not need to remove all of the skin, but make sure you take off any skin that looks black and charred. Keep any oil that is in the bowl.

Drain the sheets of lasagne. Put 3 sheets of the lasagne in a layer on the bottom of the ovenproof dish. Spoon on a third of the tomato mixture. On top of this arrange the courgettes is an even layer and then spoon on another third of the tomato mixture on top.

Put 3 sheets of lasagne on top of this and then add the

roasted red peppers. Pour on any oil that is in the bowl. Spoon on the last of the tomato mixture and put the last 3 sheets of lasagne on top.

Use a hand blender to mix the tofu with the pesto, egg, milk and 2 tablespoons of the grated parmesan. Pour this on top. Cover with foil and bake for 30 minutes at 200°C/ 400°F/Gas 5. Remove the foil and sprinkle on the remaining tablespoon of grated parmesan and cook for another 10 minutes.

The Humble Potato

Why?

Over the years potatoes have received quite a bad press but are they as bad as people make out? After all they have been around for thousands of years and they are a staple food for millions of people. Like rice they contain a large amount of glycemic starch. However, as with rice and pasta, you can transform some of this glycemic starch into resistant starch and make potatoes a much healthier food to eat.

How?

Cooking and eating potatoes with their skin on retains most of the insoluble fibre they contain and this slows down the rate at which they are digested. The skin also contains most of the vitamins and minerals that are lost when the potato is peeled.

Baking and boiling potatoes and eating them straight away is not a good idea as this breaks down the starch they contain into a form that is very easy to digest. However, by cooking them and then allowing them to cool to room temperature changes some of the glycemic starch into resistant starch.

Potato, Dill Cucumber & Walnut Salad

A SALAD THAT YOU CAN EAT ON ITS OWN OR SERVE WITH FISH OR SEAFOOD. THE SALAD WILL KEEP FOR 2 DAYS IN A COVERED CONTAINER IN THE FRIDGE.

SERVES 4

6 spring onions finely sliced
450g/1lb cooked waxy salad potatoes
150g/5½oz small pickled gherkins or dill cucumbers
4 tbsp fromage frais or natural unsweetened yoghurt
60g/2¼oz pecan nuts or walnuts coarsely chopped
Hand full of parsley, chervil or dill finely chopped

Either cut the cooked potatoes into ½ cm/¼ in slices or cut them into 1cm/½ in dice. Slice the gherkins into thin rounds.

Put the yoghurt into a large bowl and add the parsley, chervil or dill, the chopped nuts and the spring onions.

Add the potatoes and the sliced gherkins. Give everything a good stir and pile it onto a serving plate.

Porcini Mushroom & Chestnut Chowder

TO MAKE THIS YOU NEED FIRM, WAXY NEW POTATOES THAT WILL NOT DISINTEGRATE WHEN
THEY ARE COOKED. YOU CAN COOK THE POTATOES THE DAY BEFORE AND STORE THEM
OVERNIGHT IN THE FRIDGE. BECAUSE OF THEIR INTENSE FLAVOUR THE PORCINI MUSHROOMS
ARE AN ESSENTIAL INGREDIENT. YOU CAN USE FROZEN, TINNED OR VACUUM PACKED
CHESTNUTS. BECAUSE OF THE POTATOES THIS SOUP WILL NOT FREEZE.

SERVES 4

3 banana shallots finely chopped
20g/¾oz Porcini mushrooms
3 tbsp olive oil
1 tsp garlic powder
½ tsp cayenne pepper
½ tsp ground turmeric
2 tsp dried rosemary finely chopped
1Kg/2 lb 4oz small waxy new potatoes cut into 5mm/¼ in slices
1.5Lt/2¼pt vegetable stock
20 peeled and cooked chestnuts cut into quarters
90g/3oz finely grated parmesan
Crushed black pepper
Finely chopped parsley or chervil to garnish

Cook the potatoes in plenty of water until they are just cooked. Drain them and put them to one side.

Bring the vegetable stock to the boil and add the Porcini mushrooms, the cayenne pepper, garlic powder, turmeric and rosemary. Turn off the heat and leave the mushrooms to soak for at least half an hour.

Bring the porchini mushrooms back to the boil and leave them simmering while you prepare the rest of the ingredients.

Heat the oil in a large saucepan and sauté the shallots for 2 or 3 minutes. Add the chestnuts and the vegetable stock with the Porcini mushrooms. Then add the cooked potatoes.

Bring to the boil, reduce the heat and simmer for 12 - 15 minutes until the potatoes are just tender. Turn off the heat and just before serving stir in the parmesan and black pepper. Garnish with finely chopped parsley or chervil.

Salmon or Trout with Cucumber & Potato Salsa

YOU CAN USE SALMON OR TROUT FOR THIS RECIPE. THE FISH CAN BE SERVED HOT OR COLD, EITHER AS A FILLET OR BROKEN INTO BITE SIZE PIECES. THE CUCUMBER AND POTATO SALSA WILL KEEP IN THE FRIDGE FOR 2 DAYS.

SERVES 4

4 fillets of salmon each weighing about 150g/5½oz
½ lemon thinly sliced
4 bay leaves.

FOR THE POTATO SALSA

16 - 20 small cooked new potatoes
1 large telegraph cucumber, peeled, cut in half lengthways and de-seeded
8 spring onions finely chopped
1 finely chopped green chilli
1 - 2 cloves of garlic crushed
2 tbsp capers drained and roughly chopped
1 tbsp finely chopped fresh dill
1 tbsp chopped flat leaf parsley or chervil
Finely grated zest of 2 limes
Juice of 2 limes
2 tbsp olive oil
Sprigs of fresh dill or parsley to garnish.

Pre heat the oven to 200°C/ 400°F/Gas 5

Line a small baking try with foil. Put the fillets of salmon on the foil, skin side down and tuck a bay leaf under each one. Arrange the slices of lemon on top of the fish and cover with a piece of foil. Turn over all 4 edges to seal the fish in a large parcel.

Bake the fish for 20 minutes until it is set and translucent. The precise time it takes will depend on the thickness of the fish. When the fish is cooked take it out of the oven but leave it in the foil to rest while you prepare the salsa.

Cut the potatoes and cucumber into small 5mm/¼ in dice and put them into a large bowl. Add the spring onions, chilli, garlic, capers, dill, parsley and lime zest and give everything a good stir.

Put the lime juice and olive oil into a small jar, put on the lid and give it a good shake. Mix this into the potato and cucumber.

When you are ready to serve the fish, put a small pile of the salsa onto a plate and place the fillet of fish on top. Garnish with the herbs. Alternatively you can break the fish into bite size pieces.

Pickled Herring, Sweetcorn & Potato Salad

THIS IS AN ALMOST INSTANT MEAL. YOU CAN USE BISMARK HERRINGS OR ROLL MOPS TO MAKE THE RECIPE. THESE ARE READY TO EAT AND USUALLY SOLD IN JARS OR PLASTIC TUBS. THE HERRINGS NEED TO BE STORED IN THE FRIDGE BUT AS THEY HAVE A FAIRLY LONG SHELF LIFE THEY ARE A USEFUL STORE CUPBOARD INGREDIENT. ALL YOU NEED TO DO IS DRAIN THEM BEFORE USING THEM IN THE RECIPE.

THERE ARE MANY DIFFERENT WAYS OF SERVING OILY FISH LIKE HERRINGS, MACKEREL AND SARDINES THAT HAVE BEEN PRESERVED. THIS RECIPE USES COLD POTATOES BUT YOU COULD USE CANNELLINI BEANS AS AN ALTERNATIVE.

SERVES 4

Large 500g/1lb 2oz jar Bismark Herring or Roll Mops
1 small red onion finely sliced
700g/1 lb 9oz cooked waxy salad potatoes
100g/3½ oz small pickled gherkins
250g/9oz cooked sweetcorn kernels
Hand full of parsley, chervil or dill finely chopped
Baby salad leaves to serve

Either slice the cooked potatoes or cut them into 1cm/½ in dice. Slice the gherkins into thin rounds. Wash and drain the sweetcorn.

Put the potatoes and gherkins into a large serving dish and add the sweetcorn kernels and the sliced onion.

Cut the Bismark Herrings or Roll Mops into bite size pieces and place them on top.

Garnish with the chopped herbs and serve on a bed of baby salad leaves.

Potato Tortilla with Za'atar Spices

A SIMPLE TORTILLA THAT MAKES A REALLY GOOD MEAL OR BREAKFAST DISH. YOU WILL NEED FIRM WAXY SALAD POTATOES TO MAKE THIS.

SERVES 4

500g/1lb 2oz cooked sliced salad potatoes
2 tsp Sambol Oelek OR chilli paste
4 finely sliced spring onions
1 clove of garlic crushed
2 tsp ready made Za'atar
1 tbsp olive oil
6 large free range eggs
3 tbsp natural unsweetened yoghurt
100g/3½ oz crumbled feta

You will need a 24cm/10 in non stick frying pan or chefs pan with a lid to make this. Pre heat the oven to 180°C/350°F/Gas 4

Heat 1 tablespoon of the olive oil in a the frying pan. Add the crushed garlic and cook over a medium heat for 2 minutes. Don't let the garlic brown. Add the cooked potatoes and stir the garlic into them. Leave them to heat through while you mix the eggs.

Whisk the eggs in a large bowl with the Sambol Oelek, 1 tsp of the Za'atar and the yoghurt. Stir in the sliced spring onions.

Pour in the egg mixture over the potatoes and garlic. Cook for 5 minutes then cover the frying pan and put it into the oven. Cook for 20 minutes.

Take off the lid, add the crumbled feta and sprinkle over the remaining Za'atar spices. Cook uncovered for another 5 minutes until the centre of the tortilla is just set and the cheese is lightly brown.

Za'atar

A MIXTURE OF HERBS AND SPICES THAT IS WIDELY USED IN THE MIDDLE EAST AS A SPRINKLE FOR SALADS AND VEGETABLES. ZA'ATAR IS WIDELY AVAILABLE IN SUPERMARKETS BUT YOU CAN MAKE YOUR OWN. STORE ZA'ATAR IN AN AIRTIGHT CONTAINER.

2 tsp dried oregano
1 tsp sumac
3 tsp toasted sesame seeds
1 tsp ground cumin
Pinch chilli flakes or Cayenne pepper
½ tsp dried garlic granules (optional)
¼ tsp salt flakes

Put everything into a blender, spice grinder or pestle and mortar and process until about half of the sesame seeds have been crushed. Add the sea salt crystals and give them a quick whiz to mix everything together and break down the crystals.

Meat

Why?

There is no doubt that meat is a highly nutritious food and it is clearly an important part of our diet. A 100 gram pork chop contains 75 gram of water, 20 grams of protein, 1.8 grams of monounsaturated fat, 1.5 grams of saturated fat and 0.5 grams of polyunsaturated fat. Despite the horror stories about saturated fat most meat has more unsaturated fat than saturated fat. Just like nuts and other natural unprocessed food these fats are put together by nature in more or less the right proportions. It is only when we start messing around with meat and adding tenderising chemicals, dyes, browning agents in the form of sugar and then wrapping it up in breadcrumbs and frying it in vegetable oil that things start to go wrong.

Most of us eating a typical western diet eat meat at least once a day but studies of our early ancestors and the hunter gatherers that are left in their natural environment show that only about 30% of their daily calories come from meat.

Notwithstanding any potential health risks of eating meat there are other reasons why reducing the amount of meat we eat is a good idea. Unless we go out of our way to find certified 'organic' grass fed meat, almost all of the meat we buy in supermarkets and food stores comes from animals and poultry that have been intensively reared. This means that the animals have been fed on grain, soya or corn and their diet supplemented with hormones and antibiotics that pass through into the meat. Both the amount and type of fat in the meat of animals that have been intensively reared is very different to that found in 'natural' meat. In particular the amount of Omega 6 is far higher than in grass fed meat and this makes meat from intensively reared animals a highly inflammatory food to eat. When you add to all this the environmental cost of all types of meat production, it is clear that we all need to reduce the amount of meat we are eating.

How?

Avoid processed meats because they all contain preservatives and high levels of sodium. Try to reduce the number of times you eat meat to two or three times and week and eat it in smaller amounts. Start experimenting with offal and the cheaper cuts of meat. Adding cooked pulses to meat dishes will add some additional protein, 'pad out' the meat and make it go farther.

Chocolate & Cocoa

Or rather the dark, bitter 85% plus cocoa solid chocolate with no sugar. Most definitely not the 50% or less cocoa solid chocolate 'candy' bar that is packed full of sugar, vegetable oils, trans fats and loads of other things that are definitely not good for you. This type of confectionery makes you ill as well as fat.

Why?

High quality cocoa powder and high cocoa mass chocolate without sugar are very healthy things to eat. But, and its a very big but, not all chocolate and cocoa powder are created equal. The word chocolate really does mean the 85% plus stuff with little or no sugar and to most of us it tastes quite bitter. This type of chocolate is a potent source of antioxidants and it is rich in the polyphenols and flavonoids that help reduce inflammation. Depending on the way it is processed cocoa can contain up to 10% of its weight in flavonoids. The flavonoid group contains the same catechins, epicatechins and proanthocyanidins that are found in green and white tea.

Chocolate is made from seeds or beans that are formed inside pods of fruit on a plant called Theobroma Cacao, or "Food of the Gods", that is native to Central and South America. It has been used as a drink by the indigenous population of South America for hundreds of years, and this drink was known for its health giving properties. However, this drink is very different to the cocoa drink we know today.

The beans of the cacao tree are extremely bitter, in fact they are so bitter they are inedible. Before they are made into chocolate they go through a process of fermentation, sprouting, drying, cleaning and roasting that brings out their flavour. At the end of this process they are ground and the cocoa butter they contain extracted and sold as a separate product. Around 55% of the cocoa bean is cocoa butter. Like olive oil this contains oleic acid and a high proportion of saturated fats that are derived from stearic and palmitic acids. Unlike the cocoa mass, the cocoa butter contains very few flavonoids. The cocoa mass or cocoa powder that is left after the cocoa butter is removed is what we know as cocoa. With most of the chocolate we eat, other fats and oils that are not particularly healthy are put back into the cocoa mass together with sugar, milk, bulking agents and flavouring. In 'healthy' chocolate the cocoa butter is put back in with just enough sugar to make the chocolate edible.

As with all things that are heated the flavonoids and antioxidants in the cocoa beans are damaged during the roasting process. Most chocolate is heated to very high temperatures, so not only are the flavonoids and antioxidants significantly reduced in numbers, other damage causing substances like Advanced Glycation End products are also produced. However, some companies process cocoa slowly at low temperatures and in a way that retains many of the health giving benefits of the chocolate.

How?

The first thing is to find a good source of healthy chocolate or sugar free cocoa powder and this is easier said than done. Medicinal grade chocolate or high quality baking chocolate or cocoa is an option but as this is very difficult to come by most of us have to be pragmatic and make compromises. Go for 85% plus cocoa solids with little or no added sugar. When it comes to chocolate you get what you pay for, the more expensive, generally the higher the quality. If you have access to the internet go online and see what you can find.

Chocolate Brownies

USE ANY TYPE OF NUT TO MAKE THESE, ALMONDS, PECAN NUTS, HAZELNUTS AND WALNUTS ALL WORK. YOU CAN SERVE THE BROWNIES ON THEIR OWN OR WITH FROMAGE FRAIS. YOU WILL NEED A 20CM OR 8 IN SQUARE CAKE TIN.

Makes 12 – 16
100g/3½oz nuts
100g/3½oz butter
100g/3½oz 70% or 85% cocoa solids chocolate
2 large free range eggs beaten
40g/1½ oz wholegrain spelt
40g/1½ oz polenta
3 tbsp dark unrefined Muscavado sugar
2 tsp baking powder

Pre heat the oven to 180°C/ 350°F/Gas 4 and grease and line the cake tin.

Roughly chop the nuts and toast them for 4 minutes. Take them out and give them a stir, put them back in and toast them for another 4 minutes. Take them out of the oven and put them to one side while you prepare other ingredients.

Turn the oven down to160°C/ 325°F/Gas 3.

Break the chocolate into a dry bowl, add the butter and sugar and put the bowl over a saucepan of gently simmering water until the chocolate and butter have melted. Stir until the mixture is smooth. Turn off the heat.

Put the spelt, polenta, baking powder and nuts into a bowl. Add the melted chocolate and the beaten eggs and mix well. Spoon into the prepared tin, smooth over the surface and bake for 25 - 30 minutes. The brownies will feel slightly springy in the middle when they are cooked.

Leave to cool before cutting into 12 or 16 pieces.

Chocolate Crunch Biscuits

THIS RECIPE IS A WAR TIME RECIPE THAT USES NO EGG AND VERY LITTLE SUGAR AND FAT. THE BISCUITS ARE VERY EASY TO MAKE.

Make about 16

2 heaped tbsp unrefined dark Muscavado sugar
2 tbsp cocoa powder
50g/1¾oz butter
3 tbsp water
½ tsp vanilla extract (optional)
150g/5½oz flaked oatmeal

You will need a 20cm/8 in square tin, preferably silicon bakeware, .

Pre heat the oven to 160°C/ 325°F/Gas 3. If the baking tin you are using is metal grease the bottom of the tin really well or line it with baking parchment.

Put the butter, sugar, water and cocoa powder into a medium size saucepan and melt the butter over a gentle heat. Stir it well to remove any lumps of sugar and cook, stirring once or twice over a very low heat to 'cook' the cocoa powder and remove the raw cocoa taste.

Turn off the heat and add the flaked oatmeal to the butter and cocoa. Mix thoroughly. The mix will be quite dry and become harder to work as it cools. Put it into the prepared tin and using the back of a spoon press it down firmly.

Cook for 20 minutes until it is firm to touch. Take it out of the oven and put to one side to cool a little.

When it is cool enough to handle put the biscuit onto a chopping board and use a sharp knife to cut it into 16 pieces.

Red wine

Why?

Red wine as part of a healthy diet! Like sugar, our love affair with alcohol goes back a long way. Man has consumed alcohol in various forms for thousands of years. Even primitive man unknowingly consumed it when he ate fruit that was partially fermented.

All alcoholic drinks, irrespective of whether they are beer, lager, wine or spirits contain ethanol and ethanol is the only type of alcohol that we can consume. We have developed the enzymes needed to digest it but we have not developed the enzymes needed to digest other types of alcohol. Ethanol is metabolised by our liver in more or less the same way as fructose. It is very quickly converted into glycogen and if the glycogen stores in our liver are full the glycogen is quickly converted into fat and stored in fat cells. In addition to ethanol all alcoholic drinks contain carbohydrates usually in the form of sugar, some more than others, and when we digest the sugar and convert it into glucose we need to produce insulin to regulate it. Too much sugar means too much glucose and excess glucose is converted into glycogen and this ultimately ends up as fat.

When we consume alcohol it can interfere with our body's normal antioxidant defence mechanisms because it strips our body of some of its Vitamin C and some of the essential trace elements and micro nutrients it needs to make its own antioxidants. Zinc is of particular interest here as alcohol increases the amount of zinc that is excreted, so consuming alcohol on a regular basis, especially if it is consumed in relatively large amounts, can potentially lead to low levels of zinc or in extreme cases zinc deficiency.

So the message is that alcohol is not very good for us and drinking it is basically not a good idea. Or is it? As with most things all sources of alcohol are not created equal. When consumed as part of a meal red wine appears to slow down the digestion of the meal and this results in more stable blood glucose levels. Because of this, red wine is the key element in what is often described as the 'French Paradox'; the consumption of a rich and potentially unhealthy diet that appears to be made healthy by the inclusion of moderate amounts of red wine. How can red wine make an unhealthy diet healthy? Opinions differ but red wine is known to contain a group of powerful antioxidants in the form of compounds called polyphenols and these appear to have a beneficial effect on our health.

Resveratrol is just one of many polyphenol compounds and it is attracting a great deal of attention at the moment as it is known to be a powerful sirtuin regulator. Hence the inclusion of red wine in The Sirt Food diet. As well as red skinned fruit and vegetables in general, resveratrol is found in large amounts in the skin of red grapes. So the theory is that drinking moderate amounts of red wine, especially with a meal, will provide you with a supply of resveratrol that will mop up some free radicals, encourage your cells to go into 'repair' mode and up regulate your metabolism by improving your insulin response.

When ever you read about diet and health the consumption of alcohol is invariably a hot topic and sorting out fact from fiction or wishful thinking is not easy. Can we trust the health advice we are given on drinking? Well the answer is, it depends on when the advice was given and on where you live. In 1979 the UK government advised men to drink no more than 56 units of alcohol a week. This was later reduced to 36 units, then to 28 units and then to 21 units. In 2016 the figure was reduced further to 14 units, this time for both men and women. Current guidelines for a man in Spain are 35 units of alcohol a week, in Denmark and Ireland 21 units and in America 25 units, but in America the recommendation for women is half of this, just over 12 units. In the UK, when the chief medical officer announced the new guidelines she asserted that there is no safe level of drinking and that the health benefits of moderate alcohol consumption were "old wives tales". This is interesting as the evidence is actually quite the opposite. The health benefits of moderate drinking are clear to see when you look at the data and because 'booze' generally is such a contentious issue the data is very robust. In 2016 just after the new guidelines were issued in the UK the US National Institute on Alcohol Abuse and Alcoholism published a review that maintained their previous guidelines for men of 25 units a week. They also stated that in their opinion 26,000 deaths from heart disease, diabetes and stroke a year were prevented by the moderate consumption of alcohol.

There is no "one size fits all solution" and alcohol consumption will always be a personal issue, but one thing that you need to be mindful of is that alcohol weakens your will power, so once you have had one drink it is easy to have another and before you know it you start snacking, usually on the type of food that is not good for you. When you look at the facts red wine does contain some powerful antioxidants and it does appear to offer some protection against heart disease, stroke and some cancers, so the general consensus is that a little red wine could actually be good for you. Just remember to drink sensibly.

Never Eat

Polyunsaturated Vegetable Oils & Trans Fats

Sunflower, safflower, canola, peanut, corn, soya and rapeseed oils as well as margarine and low fat spreads.

Why?

Because they are major sources of highly reactive free radicals that have the potential to severely damage your health. They also contribute to a major imbalance between the Omega 3 and Omega 6 Essential Fatty Acids and this makes them highly inflammatory. In fact the amount of Omega 6 consumed in a typical Western Diet can make inflammation run out of control. Hot pressed polyunsaturated vegetable oils are totally man made products and they are most definitely not good for you.

Ask yourself how much convenience food you consume in a day. In a typical Western diet about 30% of our daily calories from polyunsaturated vegetable oils and most of these are hidden in convenience foods. The polyunsaturated vegetable oils are incorporated into cell membranes where they wreak havoc, disrupting the cell's metabolism and ultimately damaging or killing the cell. When this happens free radicals are released into the blood stream, resulting in increased pressure on your body's antioxidant defences and ultimately oxidative stress sets in. Trans fats are polyunsaturated vegetable oils in their worst possible form and for many years they have been consistently linked to cardiovascular disease.

How?

Switch to butter and olive oil. They are healthy foods that have both stood the test of time. Goose fat and lard are also alternatives but use all of these in moderation. Fat is a high energy food so it contains a lot of calories; just 8 grams of butter contains 50 kcal and 1 tablespoon olive oil contains 120 kcal. If you want to use salad dressings make your own using olive oil. When you buy any oil make sure you read the label carefully and preferably buy oils that have been 'cold pressed'. Oil that is in a dark bottle is best as it protects the oil from sunlight and also keep the oil in the fridge as this also reduces the rate at which it oxidises.

A note about labelling legislation as this varies enormously between countries. In the EU cold pressed means just that, but in many other countries labels are simply marketing tools that can say more or less anything.

Which foods contain polyunsaturated oils and trans fats?

In terms of trans fats we are back to the old chestnut of biscuits, cookies, cakes, more or less anything that is processed, as well as margarines, 'spreadable' butter and non dairy creamers. The number of products containing polyunsaturated vegetable oils is enormous; crisps, chips, fries, salad dressings, mayonnaise, anything that is fried commercially. It really is staggering how these unhealthy oils have stealthily found their way into our food and even more staggering how they are so often presented as 'the healthy' option.

Sugar

Why:

Because your body simply does not need sugar, irrespective of what form it comes in. It can make all the glucose it needs from the carbohydrates you consume, even when you have reduced your carbohydrate intake and changed from refined carbohydrates to unrefined whole grains. All consuming sugar will do is increase your insulin sensitivity and contribute to a few extra pounds in body weight.

How:

Cutting out sugar is easier said than done especially if you eat a lot of convenience foods and you drink a lot of non diet soft drinks. The difficult thing about cutting out sugar is that so many foods contain it; ice cream, mayonnaise and salad dressings are loaded with it and even 'ready meals' and TV diners have it added in one form or another as a browning agent. In fact sugar is used in more or less all processed foods as a preservative. There is no easy solution to cutting out sugar. It is not easy but there are some very good web sites that can help. You are either going to have to stop consuming the types of food that contains or start making your own, without sugar.

Tips:

- Substitute fizzy water for carbonated soft drinks. Ignore the stuff on the internet that says carbonated fizzy water is bad for you. It is yet more misinformation. Ten teaspoons of sugar in each regular can of soft drink damages your health far more than carbonated water.
- Make your own lemonade. It freezes really well and the Vitamin C is not damaged by freezing.

- Green, white and oolong teas are great and they are really good for you. In fact they form an essential part of a healthy diet.
- Read the labels on food very carefully and beware of the words 'natural' or 'no refined sugars'. Remember fructose is a natural sugar and concentrated grape extract is still sugar.
- Be wary of anything in a box or packet with a long shelf life as it is likely that sugar will have been used as a preservative.

Refined Carbohydrates

Why?

Refined carbohydrates are impoverished foods that have had many of their essential nutrients removed. It is thought that primitive man consumed between 50 and 100 grams of carbohydrates a day and these would have been complex and completely unrefined. These carbohydrates would also have been obtained from tubers and different types of grains, seeds and cereals. Today, on average, most of us who eat a traditional western diet are consuming between 350 and 600 grams of refined carbohydrates each day. A massive increase that our bodies are not designed to cope with. In addition most of these carbohydrates come from wheat or rice and they are all in a highly refined form that is easily and quickly converted into sugar.

How?

When we think about carbohydrates we automatically think of bread, rice, pasta, potatoes and cakes but many packaged and processed foods contain hidden carbohydrates. Many of us eat them every day and as they have little nutritional value the best advice is to stop eating them. Switch to complex unrefined whole grain carbohydrates and foods that are made from them.

Change from white and wholemeal bread to whole grain bread, pumpernickel type rye or sour dough bread that is partially fermented before it is cooked. Better still, have a go at making your own bread using oatmeal, spelt and rye flour. It doesn't have to be yeast bread either. Soda bread is great and it only takes minutes to prepare.

Tips:

We live in a culture that expects to have a portion of carbohydrates with each meal. Most of us begin our day with a carbohydrate rich breakfast, have a carbohydrate rich morning snack followed by a carbohydrate rich lunch and then we end our day with a carbohydrate rich meal. There is no doubt that we need to eat carbohydrates but how much should we be eating?

The amount of carbohydrate we need on a daily basis depends on our age, our sex, our level of activity and our overall health. Most dietary guidelines recommend that carbohydrates make up between 45% and 65% of our daily calorie intake, so if you eat 2,000 calories a day between 900 and 1,300 calories should come from carbohydrates. This translates into between 225 grams and 325 grams which is more or less half of what most of us are thought to be consuming.

Moving away from a diet that is high in refined carbohydrates takes some doing as for many of us carbohydrates are comfort foods. Try substituting lightly cooked mashed cauliflower for rice, shredded cabbage 'tagliatelle' works well. Beans like borlotti, fava beans, chickpeas and butter beans are a great source of protein and fibre as well as carbohydrate and they contain far less carbohydrate than the same weight of potatoes, rice or pasta.

Artificial Sweeteners

Why?

We all know that going sugar free is not easy but using artificial sweeteners is not the solution. While they satisfy our cravings for sweet things they are man made products that are potentially toxic. They can damage our health and all the evidence shows that in the long term rather than reduce the number of calories we consume they actually increase the number of calories we consume.

There is plenty of evidence out there that tells us that artificial sweeteners are not a good idea. It is an undisputed fact that the weight and Body Mass Index of people who consume low calorie 'diet' drinks on a regular basis is consistently higher than the BMI of people who do not drink regular or diet drinks. But making bad food choices and consuming extra calories is not the only reason why this happens. It would appear that artificial sweeteners favour the growth of certain types of bacteria in our digestive tract. These bacteria are able in some way to extract extra energy from the food we eat so from a given meal they make more calories available to us. Ultimately these extra calories end up as fat and a higher BMI.

Fruit Juice and Smoothies

Why?

The commercial fruit juice and smoothies that you buy in the Supermarket contain enormous amounts of sugar as well as preservatives, flavouring and colouring agents and they are devoid of fibre. They are not a healthy way to start your day.

How.

Eat whole fruit instead of fruit juice, apples, oranges, cranberries, anything the fruit juice is made from. You will be getting the full benefit of the fruit as well as the fibre. There is an old saying that if you are not hungry enough to eat an apple then you are not hungry. You will get far more satisfaction from the 'crunch factor' of one apple than drinking a glass of apple juice that contains the sugar equivalent of three or four apples and no fibre.

In terms of smoothies buy a small blender and make your own. Use fruit and natural unsweetened yoghurt and where ever possible use the whole fruit. Smoothies freeze really well so make them in large quantities and take them out of the freezer when you need them.

Fried, Grilled & Roasted Food

Why?

Frying food at high temperatures, especially in polyunsaturated vegetable oils produces large amounts of free radicals. But even without oil, cooking at high temperatures can produce some highly damaging substances, such as Advanced Glycation End products or glycotoxins. These are known to be one of the primary factors in degenerative diseases and premature ageing. Not only do Advanced Glycation End products give rise to inflammation, they also damage cells and increase oxidative stress.

Advanced Glycation End products are created when sugars interact with proteins. Our bodies make their own AGE's, the higher the blood sugar level the more AGE's we make, and this explains why scientists studying diabetes have known about them for many years. Advanced Glycation End products also come from food and around 10% of the AGE's in our food are absorbed. As only about 3% of these are excreted, over time the levels of AGE's in our body slowly build up.

How

Different foods produce different amounts of AGE's and different cooking methods also give rise to different amounts. Frying, roasting and grilling create the most, whereas boiling, steaming and braising the least. High protein meats, poultry and fish create more than vegetables although chips and fries also contain them.

How many AGE's are we consuming? It is thought that the standard American diet contains three times the recommended safety limit each day. The more raw foods we eat the less AGE's we consume. Interestingly, adding lemon juice or vinegar reduces the number of AGE's that form so marinading food before it is cooked is a good idea. Changing our cooking methods and eating less animal protein will reduce the amount of AGE's our bodies are exposed to. All manufactured foods contain them, even seemingly innocuous things like flaked breakfast cereals, soy sauce, flavourings and dressings.

To Summarise

Avoid:

- Packaged foods, especially those with a long list of ingredients.
- When preparing food select raw, fresh, steamed or boiled foods and avoid fried, grilled, BBQ'd and roasted foods.

Eat more:

- Vegetables and fruit; deep red, yellow, orange, green. Eat the rainbow we have all been told to eat. Vegetables and fruit provides us with vitamins, minerals, phytonutrients, fibre and antioxidants.
- Healthy fats. Include plenty of Omega 3 oils from oily fish, salmon, herring, mackerel, sardines, avocados, and olive oil and don't be afraid to eat butter.
- Fibre is one thing many of us have a shortage of in our diet. Yes,in the short term it can create flatulence but this soon passes. More important is that it creates a favourable environment for healthy bacteria to live in.
- Herbs and spices; parsley, chervil, basil, coriander, garlic, ginger, turmeric. It is a long list. They all contain antioxidants and anti-inflammatory components. The amount they contain may be small but every little helps to make a healthy diet.

Eliminate:

- Polyunsaturated vegetable oils. Any potential health giving properties have been removed during processing and they are overloaded with Omega 6 fats that fuel inflammation.
- Trans Fats and hydrogenated fats. Our bodies have no means of using them and they are a major source of free radicals and inflammation that are known to increase the risk of coronary heart disease. Together with polyunsaturated vegetable oils they are the single most damaging food in our modern Western Diet.
- Refined and processed carbohydrates; bread, pastries, cakes, biscuits, fruit juice are all rapidly digested and lead to rapid rises in blood glucose levels that create insulin spikes.
- Artificial sweeteners and preservatives. They have no nutritional value and they ultimately lead to increased weight and a higher BMI.

Some thoughts to help you on your way

Be suspicious about food that is advertised on TV.

Most advertising is for processed foods and most processed foods contain additives, usually in the form of sugar and salt. The food manufacturers are spending a lot of money on the advertising and are looking for big returns on their products. This means big profits. They are always one step ahead of the game, so if you buy food that is advertised it is unlikely to be good for you.

Eat when you are hungry - not because you are bored.

Ask yourself why you are eating and whether you are really hungry.

Understand the difference between thirst and hunger.

Have a drink of water or make some tea before you reach for something to eat or snack on.

Do all of your eating at a table.

Don't eat while you are working at a desk, walking around or watching TV. Why? Because when we do this we eat mindlessly and therefore eat more. If you do eat when you are not sitting at the table, eat fruit, vegetables and a few nuts, not chips, crisps, biscuits, cakes and burgers.

Reduce the size of your plate !!
Stop eating BEFORE you feel full.

Most of the long lived people in the world stop eating when they are about 80% full.

Don't go to the supermarket to do your shopping when you are hungry.

If you do, you are more likely to buy fast food, junk food and convenience foods. The bakery counter near the entrance may become irresistible.

Carry a magnifying glass with you when you go shopping.

If you do need to read labels remember that they are part of the marketing process. The ingredients listed on labels are there to comply with the law, they are not there to provide you with information. Ingredients are always difficult to read as they are invariably in very small print.

Real food does not come in packets and it does not need a nutritional label.

If you do buy packaged foods read the label carefully.

Contents are often disguised. Maltose and dextrose are still sugar, maltodextrin is still starch and 'enriched' usually means that most of the good things have been taken out and a few 'not so good' things put back in. Real food does not need to be 'enriched'.

Cook from scratch as often as you can.

There are hidden additives, trans fats and sugar in almost all of the processed and ready-to-eat foods that we don't normally think contain them.

Convenience foods.

It is impossible to break the habits of a lifetime so eat all the convenience foods you want provided you make them yourself. There's nothing wrong with eating fried foods, pastries and ice cream once in a while but manufacturers have made it easy and cheap for us to eat them every day. If you have to make them yourself you will eat them far less often and you certainly won't eat them every day.

If you can buy something for less than the cost of making it yourself there is a reason.

Packaged, processed and convenience foods disguise cheap, low quality ingredients, things that are simply not good to eat.

Eating is a social activity.

Try not to eat alone. The more you interact with your fellow diners the less you will eat.

Learn to cook. It can be an exciting adventure that can give you a lot of pleasure

Appendix

The Kitchen & The Store Cupboard

Cooking at home requires some advance planning and preparation. If you do not already 'cook' here are some tips on how to begin.

Kitchen Equipment

A well equipped kitchen saves time and effort and it can take much of the drudgery out of the preparation of food. Kitchen tools and equipment come in a many different options, ranging from basic and manual to fully automatic with all the bells and whistles.

You know the basics; sharp knives, cutting boards, spatulas, pots and pans, measuring cups and spoons etc. but there are other tools and appliances that are 'nice to have' rather than essential. Here are a few of our favorite 'essential' kitchen tools that will make life in the kitchen that much easier.

A Handheld (stick) Blender

With chopping/blending and whisk attachments. You can use this to blend soup, purée and whiz ingredients together and whisk egg whites.

A Food Processor

For slicing, grating, chopping and general mixing. You may be able to manage quite well with only a very small one but you will find a machine with a 2½ **Litre/4¼ pint/**10 cup bowl the most useful.

Blender

If you feel unable to stretch to a food processor a small blender will help with some of the chopping and blending tasks.

Coffee Grinder:

Reserved for grinding spices as spices taste much better when they are freshly ground.

Pestle and Mortar

As an alternative for grinding spices and making pestos.

Silicon Bakeware

I am a great convert to silicon bakeware so if you have not already invested in conventional baking tins buy some silicon baking equipment As a suggestion it is worth investing in

- 1.4Lt/2½ pt loaf tin,
- 20cm/8 in square cake tin,
- 24cm/10 in diameter round cake tin,
- 150ml/5 fl oz (¼ pt) muffin tins and
- silicon baking mat.

A Potato Ricer

Not strictly essential but useful as it 'mashes' things without turning them into a mush.

Cooking Pans

You will find a non stick 24cm/10in frying pan or chef's pan (with a lid) that can go in the oven as well as on the hob, a wok and some non stick saucepans are very useful.

The Store Cupboard

For most of us, whether it is because of convenience or simple economics, shopping in supermarkets is an inevitable part of our life. As well as fruit and vegetables they are a good place to stock up on canned and frozen food and the things you need to buy in large quantities. Farmers markets, speciality markets, ethnic markets and on line retailers often carry the harder to find ingredients that your local supermarkets does not stock. Whatever you buy and wherever you buy it remember to read the labels so that you know exactly what is in the food you are buying. If you can find the time, grow some things yourself, especially herbs and sprouting seeds like mustard cress and alfalfa. You don't need a lot of land - pots take up very little space and nothing tastes better than something you have grown yourself.

In addition to fresh ingredients you need a well stocked pantry. Don't forget the freezer. Here is a list of some of the ingredients you will need to have on hand as you cook your way through the recipes in this book.

Herbs:

Most fresh herbs will keep in the fridge for up to a week if they are wrapped in kitchen paper and stored in a box. They also keep well in a jar of water on the window sill. Better still, buy growing herbs. Basil, parsley and coriander do well in pots and a small bay plant on the window sill is very useful. Herbs also freeze well - see the recipes for making different types of pesto, and freezing herbs does not affect their nutritional value. Making your own pesto and keeping a supply in the freezer is well worth the effort. Drying herbs is another option but with the exception of dill and rosemary, most dried herbs just don't taste the same as fresh ones.

Because they have powerful anti-inflammatory properties the recipes in this book use a lot of ginger and chilli. You can buy frozen grated ginger and frozen chopped chilli. As with different types of pesto you will find a stock of this in the freezer very useful.

Spices:

It is best to buy whole spices as once they are ground they begin to loose their flavour quickly. A coffee grinder reserved for spices works well or you can use a simple pestle and mortar. Whether they are whole or ground, store spices away from heat, light and moisture and replace them every six months. A list of some of the less common spices that you need to look out for:-

Tamarind: used extensively in Asian cooking. It gives food a characteristic tart, sour flavour.

Sumac: a Middle Eastern spice with a sharp slightly sour taste.

Chilli: as well as whole fresh chillies you can use chilli as a paste, ground into a fine powder or very finely chopped as in Sambol Oelek.

Turmeric: This has very strong anti-inflammatory properties.. If you are lucky enough to be able to buy this fresh do so, otherwise you will need to rely on dried powdered turmeric.

Garam Masala: A useful Asian blend of spices.

Garlic: Another strongly anti-inflammatory ingredient. As well as fresh garlic, stock up on dried garlic granules and if you an find them some smoked dried garlic granules.

Healthy fats and oils:

Make sure you have a supply of healthy fats and oils; cold pressed olive oil, butter and, if you can buy it, clarified butter or Ghee. Store the olive oil in the dark or in the fridge to slow down the rate at which it oxidises.

Miscellaneous Ingredients

- Wholegrain Spelt. An 'old' type of grain that is the same family as wheat. It contains less gluten than wheat and is a healthy alternative to conventional whole grain flour.
- Flaked and fine oatmeal. You can usually find flaked or rolled oats in your local supermarket but fine oatmeal, sometimes referred to as pin head oatmeal, is more difficult to obtain. You can make your own by processing a batch of flaked oats in a blender or food processor until the oats look like a coarse flour. Store the fine oatmeal in an airtight jar.
- Dried Porchini mushrooms or dried Ceps.
- Truffle oil, an expensive luxury that is well worth the investment.
- Preserved lemons; used in Middle Eastern and North African cooking. Use lemon rind soaked for half and hour in brine if you are unable to get them.
- Miso paste: either as white miso or brown miso and used extensively in Japanese cooking, If has a strong fermented taste.
- Thai Fish Sauce. It contains a lot of salt but if you are not otherwise adding salt to your cooking, once in a while it is OK.
- Sesame Oil.
- Vegetable stock cubes or vegetable stock powder.
- Tahini, a paste made from ground sesame seeds.
- Japanese Panko Breadcrumbs; yes they are made from wheat but they are very useful when used in small amounts.

Reading Recipes

If you are new to cooking start by reading all the way through a recipe before you begin making it. Don't be put off by a long list of ingredients. A long list of ingredients does not necessarily mean that a recipe is going to be difficult.

Make sure you give yourself enough time to cook without feeling pressured or rushed. Being stressed about cooking is counter productive. As you gain experience and confidence in the kitchen you will be amazed at how quickly you can get a meal cooked and on the table. Be prepared for some things not to turn out as you expected and for some recipes not to be to your liking. The more you cook the more comfortable you will become and the more confident you will be with changing recipes to suit your personal taste. Remember, a recipe is a guide not a rigid process.

Recipe Index

Index

..

www.ingramcontent.com/pod-product-compliance
Lightning Source LLC
Chambersburg PA
CBHW081144020426
42333CB00021B/2659